Praise for Alexis Dupree

5-Star Review of
Knee Replacement Advice, Checklists, and Journal

Knee Replacement Advice, Checklists, and Journal: 5 Steps for Successful Recovery Even If You Have Complications: Practical Advice from a Patient by Alexis Dupree is a useful guide that provides practical advice from a patient's point of view on how to prepare for and recover from knee replacement surgery, even if there are complications. The book discusses the key factors about knee replacement surgery, how to prepare for the surgery and recovery, how to adopt the right attitude, to do the right thing, and living with the new knee. There is no magical solution in this book about surviving and recovering from the surgery, but it helps one to prepare and recover.

The author handles the topic extensively and methodically and shows how the surgery has helped her to maintain a reasonable quality of life. It will encourage patients and keep them motivated before going for surgery. The book gives a lot of positive messages to patients and teaches them to be survivors and adopt the right attitude. The author's personal advice and tips are helpful and can be tried out during the recovery phase. It is a must-have for all those who are planning to undergo knee replacement surgery, chiropractors, massage therapists, physical therapists, and everyone dealing with a knee replacement patient. The techniques to take care of the body after surgery are helpful and will help patients live happily with their new knee. The book gives awareness and hope to all patients recovering from surgery and to all those who are going to have knee replacement surgery.

—*Mamta Madhavan for Readers' Favorite*

… a humorous but accurate depiction of the trials and triumphs of knee replacement surgery and living with your new knee.

—*Pat Ercole, Physical Therapist*

Knee Replacement Advice, Checklists, and Journal

5 steps *for successful* recovery even if you have complications

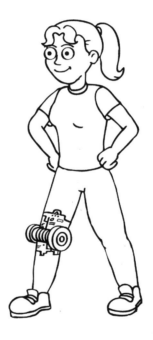

Practical Advice from a Patient

Alexis Dupree

For information about permission to reproduce selections from this book, write to Permissions, Gettier Group, LLC, 21348 Small Branch Place, Broadlands, VA 20148.

First Edition
Printed in the United States of America by Gettier Group LLC

ISBN 978-0-9860882-7-8 (trade paper)
10 9 8 7 6 5 4 3 2 1

Disclaimer
The information provided in this book is designed to provide helpful information on preparing for and recovering from knee replacement surgery from **a patient's point of view**. This book is not meant to be used nor should it be used to diagnose or treat any medical condition. For diagnosis or treatment of any medical problem, consult your own physician or surgeon. The publisher and author are not responsible for any specific health or allergy needs that may require medical supervision and are not liable for any damages or negative consequences from any treatment, action, application, or preparation, to any person reading or following the information in this book. References are provided for informational purposes only and do not constitute endorsement of any websites or other sources. Readers should be aware that the websites listed in this book may change.

Never, never, never give up.
Winston Churchill

Contents

Step 3

Adopt the Right Attitude 31

Step 4

Do the Right Thing 37

Step 5

Live with Your New Knee 49

Appendix A Checklists 55

Appendix B Recovery Journal 77

Acknowledgments

I would like to thank the following people for their helpful suggestions and comments on this book: physical therapists, Pat Ercole and Nancy McGuire, as well as Jackie Christieson, Vickie Hartman DiSanto, Carla Gladstone, Judi Hardin, Colin Helmer, Mariann Reddy, Tina Rosenthal, Victoria Sale, Judy Schramm, Karen Smith, Howard Solomon, Sharon K. Solomon, Janet Stollnitz, and Mary Anne Thomas.

Please note I've used Arabic numerals throughout the book in reference to units of time to make it easier to find and remember how much time is involved in various aspects associated with the surgery.

Introduction

This book provides practical advice from a **patient's point of view** on how to prepare for and recover from knee replacement surgery even if there are complications.

What Does This Book Include?

It explains in brief what I did or failed to do to prepare for the surgery and, more important, what helped me in achieving successful recovery.

- **Step 1, Become a Cyborg!**—This chapter summarizes my philosophy about knee replacement surgery and briefly explains key factors about the surgery.

- **Step 2, Prepare for Your Surgery and Recovery**—In this chapter I discuss the logistics of preparing for your surgery and recovery. It's not just schedule the surgery, show up at a particular time, and go home after it's done. To help everything go well, consider and implement these practical suggestions. Also follow the directions from your orthopedic surgeon and hospital staff exactly.

- **Step 3, Adopt the Right Attitude**—Assuming you have the right surgeon and hospital, your attitude is the most important factor in making surgeries and recovery go well. This chapter explains what I did to make my knee replacement surgery succeed.

- **Step 4, Do the Right Thing**—This chapter focuses on recovering from the surgery and on the various things I did to lessen pain. It also lists the answers to frequently asked questions about the surgery.

- **Step 5, Live with Your New Knee**—Once you have a new knee, life changes a bit. For one, your knee is spectacularly functional again. Second, travel becomes a bit different. Third, going to the dentist may require an additional step.

- **Appendix A, Checklists**—For your convenience, this appendix includes a checklist based on the content presented in this book. It provides space for you to record your research, such as the names of orthopedic surgeons, rehabilitation centers if needed, physical therapy centers, insurance information, etc.

- **Appendix B, Recovery Journal**—Use this journal to record your upcoming medical appointments, your prescribed medicines, a log of the medicines you take to avoid overdosing, and your thoughts or details about your recovery and whatever you please.

What's Not Included in This Book?

It does *not* contain detailed information about osteoarthritis or the structure of the knee. Nor does it explain how knee replacement surgery is performed since (1) there are always advances in medical techniques and procedures, (2) I am not a medical professional, and (3) you can consult your orthopedic surgeon and the many books, videos (YouTube is a great resource for such videos), and websites for such information. Make sure you consult legitimate websites and cross check information you find on the internet.

Why Did I Write This Book?

None of the information I read about the surgery beforehand explained how to deal with *all* of the difficulties I experienced in recovery. My knee replacement surgery in 2014 was my 13th surgery and the only one on the knee. Because of my previous surgeries, which included both minor and major surgeries, I thought I was prepared for this one. I wasn't entirely.

For me, the complications were my chronic diseases—relapsing-remitting multiple sclerosis (MS) and fibromyalgia. MS and fibromyalgia doubled my recovery time and greatly increased my level of pain.

Some people I met in physical therapy experienced complications from the actual surgery. I did not. Some needed to have the surgery redone. A few were unprepared because they had never had surgery before and the pain amazed them.

Because my diseases caused major problems—i.e., pain and lengthened my recovery—and because I'm no stranger to surgery, I want to share with others what helped me recover successfully.

Why Should You Read This Book?

A healthy person who doesn't have chronic diseases or other health issues may or may not experience the problems I did. However, everyone needs to prepare for the surgery. For example, there are practical logistics to consider, particularly if you live by yourself or don't have anyone to help you in the recovery process. Being healthy makes you less likely to have problems but is no guarantee. Being prepared helps you deal with whatever problems occur.

Note: The one advantage to my having had many surgeries is knowing how to make surgeries and their recovery go well.

What's the Most Important Thing about This Book?

It won't give you a magical solution for recovering from knee replacement surgery or, for that matter, any surgery. Surgery is an assault on your body. The body doesn't like—in fact, it hates—having someone, even a highly trained surgeon with impeccable credentials, take a knife and make the smallest slit. However, surgery may be exactly what you need to survive and keep your quality of life intact.

No Magic Here: This book does not contain magical advice about surviving and recovering from surgery. Recovery from any surgery is unique to each person. This book explains practical suggestions from a patient to help you prepare and recover.

This book explains how I recover from surgeries. My method involves being prepared, keeping a good attitude, avoiding depression, and reinforcing my determination to succeed. To be successful in recovering from surgery, one can whine—and I do sometimes—but one can't give up. No one likes a quitter. Neither should you.

Advice: At the very least, pretend you're determined and have a good attitude. Sometimes pretending something very hard about yourself makes it come true.

Disclaimer

The information provided in this book is designed to provide helpful information on preparing for and recovering from knee replacement surgery from **a patient's point of view**. This book is not meant to be used nor should it be used to diagnose or treat any medical condition. For diagnosis or treatment of any medical problem, consult your own physician or surgeon. The publisher and author are not responsible for any specific health or allergy needs that may require medical supervision and are not liable for any damages or negative consequences from any treatment, action, application, or preparation, to any person reading or following the information in this book. References are provided for informational purposes only and do not constitute endorsement of any websites or other sources. Readers should be aware that the websites listed in this book may change.

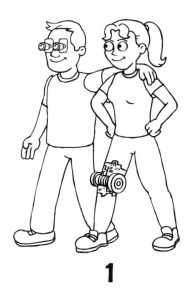

1

Become a Cyborg!

My husband and I are long-time readers of science fiction. We met at a science fiction convention 40 years ago. This chapter explains how one science fiction concept may help you in adjusting your attitude toward knee replacement surgery. It helped me.

Cyborg Nirvana

The first step when you're facing knee replacement surgery is to accept your new identity—you are about to become a cyborg! What is a cyborg, you ask? It's a person whose body contains mechanical or electrical devices and whose abilities are greater than the abilities of normal humans. Think Colonel Steve Austin (Lee Majors) in *The Six Million Dollar Man* or Jaime Sommers (Lindsay Wagner) in *The Bionic Woman.*[1] Of course, your resulting abilities won't exceed

---

1   *The Six Million Dollar Man* appeared on U.S. television from 1974–1978; *The Bionic Woman* appeared from 1976–1978. Both featured people severely crippled in accidents who received nuclear powered limbs and implants. Of course, your new knee won't be nuclear powered, but it will work far better than the crippled one you have now.

those of normal humans, but isn't it wonderful to think they might? In reality, your replaced knee becomes, with time, far more powerful than the failing and painful original one.

All Hail the Cyborg Masters!

When I was 15 years old, my right knee encountered an iron post in a sledding accident. The post didn't break any bones, but it left an enormous raised bruise on my right thigh that hung around for 3 weeks. In my late 30s, I gained weight. These factors, as well as genetics and bad luck, led to osteoarthritis in both knees. When my husband and I toured a mansion one weekend in 2013, pain in my right knee became excruciating.

That year and part of the next I received occasional cortisone shots, did physical therapy exercises, and walked in the pool in preparation for knee replacement surgery. On June 10, 2014, I became the proud recipient of a new knee joint in my right leg.

In 2015 my husband received new lenses in both his eyes during cataract surgeries. My new knee joint obliterated the pain I experienced from osteoarthritis, and my husband's vision improved dramatically. Instead of wearing Coke-bottle lenses, he sported new glasses whose weight no longer looked like they supported the entire soda industry. Although my vision was not quite as bad as his was, I envied his ability to read email on his cell phone without wearing glasses.

After my husband's surgeries, a friend posted the following comment on Facebook: "Have you considered that, with your artificial knee and your husband's artificial eyes, you're both becoming cyborgs?" My husband's comment explains why I love him: "All hail the new cyborg masters!" We are both far better than we were before.

The Miracle of Knee Surgery

Osteoarthritis is no fun, even if you're someone whose threshold for pain is great; i.e., if you experience less pain than others do. The level of pain from my failing right knee stunned me. During the year before my surgery, I willingly volunteered to receive trigger point injections[2] in my knee twice a week and cortisone shots when necessary, all in order to avoid the knee pain.

Deciding to have surgery is a big decision. Surgery isn't something to do for fun. One has surgery because it's necessary to either keep living or to maintain a reasonable quality of life.

The Decision Is Yours: You're the one who must decide when to have surgery, i.e., when the knee pain is so bad that surgery seems the only option to avoid being permanently crippled.

Only you know your own body and its reactions to medications and anesthesia. Consult your orthopedic surgeon and your primary care physician. There may be valid medical reasons for not having knee replacement surgery.

Surgery Isn't the End of the World

If you're waffling and there aren't medical reasons against having surgery, consider what the alternative to surgery entails:

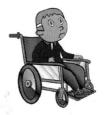

- **Experiencing excruciating pain**—Do you want to continue living with the level of pain you already have? If the level is as wretched as mine was, then choose surgery.

- **Being confined to a wheelchair sooner or later**—If you're in a wheelchair because of the pain, then surgery is the right choice.

---

2   The ingredients in the trigger point injections were all natural anti-inflammatory herbs, with a very small amount of Lidocaine and Kefolorac. These injections instantly helped relieve some of the pain. With these injections I didn't need to worry about exposing my body to harmful medicines, a very important point. In contrast, doctors must limit the number of cortisone shots they give patients because cortisone injections cause damage to tissues and can cause side effects. I had cortisone shots about every 6 months in my failing knee the year before the surgery, which helped alleviate the pain. Having weekly trigger point injections between the cortisone shots made a huge difference for me.

Choose wisely. Would surgery fix the problem and improve your life? Is surgery better than living in a wheelchair? Once you make the decision to have surgery, remind yourself often of why you decided to do so.

Is There Pain with Surgery?

Yes. There's always pain with any type of surgery. The amount and severity of pain depend on your body, your level of fitness, your level of preparation, coexisting conditions and diseases, your attitude and ability to deal with pain—what I call the "wimp factor," and your willingness to do the right thing:

Pain and Your Body
Some people have little pain. Some people have more. It depends on your body. Other factors, such as coexisting conditions and diseases, affect how much pain one experiences.

Important: Some people don't experience much pain with knee replacement surgery. Others have a lot. Also, a person may experience different pain levels with each knee replacement surgery.

My threshold for pain is low. I'm quite envious of folks who have a high tolerance for pain! Because I don't tolerate pain well, I take whatever medications or actions, such as calling the doctor or finding other help, as are reasonable to get rid of it. If you're the type of person who doesn't like to do what needs to be done to abolish pain, then prepare to suffer.

Remember: You only need to take pain medication for a comparatively short amount of time. You don't need to take it forever. Don't be a martyr. If you have pain, just take the medicine. Quit as soon as it's reasonable. Obviously, you don't want to become an addict.

Your Level of Fitness
In my observation, unless there were surgical complications, people who are in good physical condition seem to experience less pain. At least, they seem to recover far faster. The moral to this, of course, is to be in the best shape you can. Duh!

Exercise: Before the surgery, push yourself to exercise. It's good for minimizing the pain that osteoarthritis causes, and it's good preparation for the surgery.

Your Level of Preparation

Because I prepared for my knee replacement surgery—that is, I walked 50 laps in an indoor pool 3 times a week and did the physical therapy exercises, my range of motion both before and after the surgery was quite good. I am very proud of that, especially since I'm not physically fit. I hang my head in shame about that fact. So, if you're like me and are not in good physical shape, do the best you can anyway. Although I was still overweight when I had the surgery, I lost 23 pounds walking the pool without changing my diet.

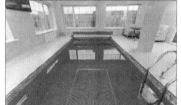

Pool Membership: Some hotels, hospitals, colleges, or recreation centers offer pool memberships. Rehabilitation pools—indoor pools filled with warm water—are wonderful for osteoarthritis. If you can afford to join a pool, find one near you. Walking in the pool is the best exercise to do for osteoarthritis.

After knee replacement surgery, the physical therapist measured the range of motion for my knee, which was quite good. It pleased me no end that my exercise at the pool produced good results despite my being overweight and unfit.

Coexisting Conditions and Diseases

Other conditions and diseases can affect the amount of pain you experience. Because of my diseases, nerve pain after the surgery haunted me for months. My recovery took twice as long as that for most folks. To be fair, my surgeon warned me that in his experience patients with MS or fibromyalgia have extra pain. I didn't really believe him. After the first month of recovery, I did.

My surgeon praised me when I saw him later. "Before the surgery I told you it would be extremely hard," he said. "But you proved me wrong. You did incredibly well." I said, "It was very difficult, but I worked very, very hard to make it successful."

Remember: Make determination your mantra. Never, never, never give up.

The Wimp Factor

The wimp factor is your attitude and ability to deal with pain. Attitude is everything. If you go into surgery expecting the worse, you

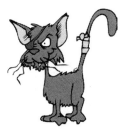

ensure a bad outcome. Instead, expect the best or, at least, expect it to be a test of your character, a test whose challenges you can master. If you found the right doctor and hospital and did the necessary preparation, have faith in yourself. Don't be a wimp. It's okay to be scared of surgery; it's stupid to think you can't handle the situation. I'm not saying don't whine occasionally. I'm saying be like the little engine that could and repeat to yourself, "The surgery will go well, the surgery will go well, the surgery will go well." Then do what you need to do during recovery to ensure it's a success.

Develop a Mantra: As I was going into surgery, I told the surgeon the mantra I was repeating to myself was "I won't be a wimp. I won't be a wimp. The surgery will be successful."

Your Willingness to Do the Right Thing

Boring as it may be, one needs to do the physical therapy exercises regularly and follow the instructions of the medical staff. If you're a maverick and don't want to comply, that's your problem. You then pay the price in pain or complications. In other words, there are consequences to what you do or fail to do.

Note: Knee replacement surgery can be quite painful for some. Don't minimize it. Do what you need to do to ensure its success.

If you miss doing an exercise, don't beat yourself up. Just do the exercise as soon as you remember. The good thing about the exercises is they *do* work. The bad thing is it seems to take forever before you feel the good results—the lessening of the pain and better functionality.

The pain disappears eventually with hard work, and your knee's functionality becomes effortless.

Bottom Line

I am very lucky. My diseases did not prevent my surgery from being successful. I worked hard, was determined, avoided depression, and expected to succeed. Recovery was lengthy, but I love my new knee and am glad I had the surgery.

If my knee replacement surgery went well, yours can, too. My motto is never, never, never give up. Look forward to being a cyborg!

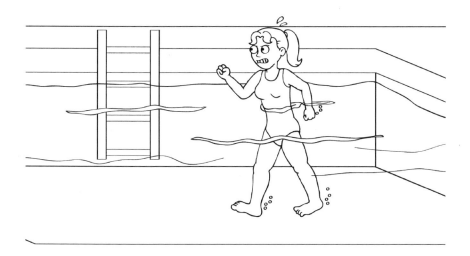

2

Prepare for Surgery and Recovery

As the patient you need to understand and prepare for the surgery and recovery and find the best surgeon possible who's covered by your medical insurance. So you need to do some research, determine where to recuperate, set up your home for your recovery, choose the right attire to wear to the hospital, and get the right equipment or tools in advance of the surgery for use during recovery.

Note: Preparing for the surgery is important, particularly if you live by yourself or don't have anyone to help you during recovery.

Do Some Research

The three areas you should research include orthopedic surgeons, the knee replacement surgery itself, and what your insurance covers.

Choose the Right Surgeon
Finding the right surgeon is imperative. This advice is true for any surgery, not just knee replacement surgery. Ways in which you can

find a good surgeon include asking for recommendations from the following:

- **Ask your primary care physician**—Ask for the names of at least two surgeons. Call their offices. Find out whether they take your 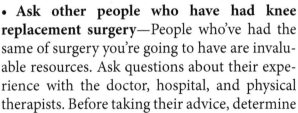 medical insurance. Meet with and evaluate them. Although it's nice to like your surgeon, liking someone doesn't mean the person is the best technically. I prefer a surgeon who knows his or her job rather than someone who is simply likable.

- **Ask nurses**—Nurses are great sources of information. They tend to recommend doctors who they know are good. After all, they work with them and observe what they do. Listen carefully to what they say.

- **Ask physical therapists**—Physical therapists may not tell you who is a bad surgeon, but they are candid about who they think is a good surgeon. Ask them for the names of the surgeons whose patients recovered well. Physical therapists are quite familiar with the problems or lack of problems their patients have after knee replacement surgery.

  - **Ask other people who have had knee replacement surgery**—People who've had the same of surgery you're going to have are invaluable resources. Ask questions about their experience with the doctor, hospital, and physical therapists. Before taking their advice, determine whether they are people whose advice you would value on other subjects. Compare different people's experiences and advice and then make your decision.

- **Check rating services**—A number of services recommend or rate doctors. Some are local services that may be found in magazines or other media; some are on the internet. These services are valuable, although I don't rate them as highly as my earlier suggestions.

Personal Experience with Rating Services: I've used several doctors who were recommended by a local rating service with mixed experiences. A couple of the listed doctors were quite fine; some were not, at least not for me. However, the orthopedic surgeon who did my knee replacement surgery is one of the doctors recommended by that service. He is quite good, and I am very happy with him. Before I checked the rating service, however, nurses and other patients had already recommended him to me.

Research the Surgery

Long before you schedule surgery, research the surgery. Good sources for research include people, books, magazines, videos, and medical sites on the internet. As a patient with chronic illnesses, I know it's important for me to educate myself about whatever the illness or ailment of the moment is. Some people prefer to have their doctors tell them what to do. However, these days it is important to be informed.

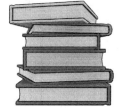

I've found YouTube to be an excellent source for information on surgeries and always consult it. Many videos on YouTube explain all aspects of knee replacement surgery. Of course, I also cross-check the information on YouTube with the information in books or medical websites.

Note: One can even watch videos of entire surgeries on YouTube. I've done that, although not everyone is willing to do so. At this point, with so many surgeries under my belt, so to speak, it doesn't bother me to watch surgeries. It helps me to be more objective about my own surgeries and not to get hyper about the whole thing. But that's just me.

Read books about joint replacement surgery. You can buy them in bookstores or online or borrow them from the local library.

Attend a Joint Replacement Class If Available

About a week before my surgery, the hospital at which it was done sponsored a mandatory hour-long class on joint replacement surgery. The class was very informative. It gave me information about how the surgery was performed in that hospital, about the room I would be in, and other details after the surgery and my recovery.

Minimally Invasive or Traditional Surgery? Someone asked me whether she should have minimally invasive or traditional surgery. That is a question for your surgeon who makes the choice based on your situation. Discuss with your surgeon the advantages and disadvantages of the types of surgeries for your specific case.

Talk to Your Insurance Company

Before the surgery, talk to your insurance company not only about

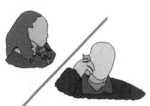 coverage for the surgery, but also about which equipment your policy covers. Equipment needed for recovery includes walkers, canes, ice machines, etc. Find out the dollar amount the insurance company pays for the various items and if there are specific companies from whom you must purchase them. Contact the providers well in advance of the surgery to make sure you can obtain the items on time.

Determine Where to Recuperate from Surgery

If you live in a house, condo, or apartment that accommodates your staying on the first floor, the best place to recuperate from the surgery is your home. If you live in a condo or apartment that's on the second, third, or higher floor with only stairs to access your home, consider arranging to stay in a rehabilitation center for the first couple of weeks after you're released from the hospital. Instead, you may be able to stay at the home of a family member or very close friend.

Note: Whether or not you're a healthy individual, you initially need assistance during the first week or so of recovery.

Because she lived in a third-floor apartment, a friend who had knee replacement surgery stayed in a rehabilitation center for the first weeks after being released from the hospital. She experienced problems with nurse's aides delivering ice for the ice machine and pain medication 45 minutes to an hour late. She contacted someone on the center's team to correct these problems.

Research rehabilitation centers in advance. Get the contact information for integral team members of the centers ahead of time so you can call the appropriate person to address any problems.

Read the following articles:

- "10 Questions to Ask When Choosing a Rehabilitation Center" by Charlotte Gerber August 12, 2016, on the verywell website (https://www.verywell.com/questions-rehabilitation-facility-1094426)

- "10 Tips for Choosing a Rehab Facility" by Bone, Muscle, and Joint Team, December 20, 2013, on the Cleveland Clinic website (https://health.clevelandclinic.org/2013/12/10-tips-for-choosing-a-rehab-facility/)

- BaylorScott&White Health, North Texas (http://www.baylorhealth.com/PHYSICIANSLOCATIONS/BIR/ABOUTUS/Pages/HowToChoose.aspx)

- "10 Questions to Ask When Selecting a Short-Term Rehab Center," May 24, 2014, Three Pillars Senior Living Communities (http://www.threepillars.org/Blog/10-Questions-to-Ask-When-Selecting-a-Short-Term-Rehab-Center.htm)

Note: Having two knee replacement surgeries at the same time is not optimal, although there may be valid reasons for doing so. If you go this route, you definitely need assistance. If you live alone, a rehabilitation center may be the only reasonable choice.

Perform These Tasks Before Surgery

Practice getting on and off of chairs and beds before surgery to make sure the ones you plan to use are of the right height. Make sure that the chairs have arms. Determine before your surgery which car is easiest for you to get in or out. It's difficult after knee replacement surgery to get in or out of a car or pickup truck that has high seats. Also, it vital to strengthen your core or arms before surgery, which means you should see a physical therapist if possible before surgery to learn appropriate exercises. Getting up from the toilet can be quite challenging. Finally, check the entrance to your home to see whether you need to make changes to enable you to enter easily after surgery or whether you need to go to a rehabilitation center for the first couple of weeks following surgery. A few steps, even a flight, are okay. More than one flight can be a problem.

Set Things Up in Advance of the Surgery

Plan in advance to have personal items and a supply of clean clothes and bed clothes easily available to you during recovery. This advice is particularly important if you don't have anyone who can assist you during recovery or if you don't want to run your caregiver ragged in doing chores you could have done before the surgery.

Advice about Caregivers: Always be cognizant of your caregiver, who is most likely a family member or friend. Being a caregiver is difficult, more difficult sometimes than being the patient. Don't take undue advantage of the person who's providing a tremendous service to you. Be smart. Accept the service when it's needed; do for yourself when you can, i.e., when you aren't going to injure yourself.

Bed

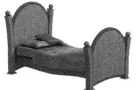

Consider the height of your bed. If it's higher than the normal height of beds, it may present problems for you when you're recovering from surgery. I slept on a sofa bed in our family room. A friend who recently had knee replacement surgery found her bed too high. She slept on a daybed.

If your bed isn't suitable and you have no other options, consider renting a hospital bed, which can be lowered or raised. Some medical insurance policies cover this expense. Ask your insurance company in advance of the surgery whether renting a hospital bed is covered.

Hospital Bed Rental: For another surgery, I determined the sofa bed would not work because it was too low. My insurance policy covered hospital beds, so I arranged for one to be delivered 3 days before the surgery. However, the company from which I ordered the bed continually made mistakes and delivered it the day *after* my surgery. This mistake was despite my calling the company every day. My husband put another mattress on top of the sofa bed mattress and I made do the first night. The point is that mistakes may happen in any company. Plan to follow up on delivery. Sometimes only one company in your area works with your insurance company; i.e., you must work with that company. Schedule delivery well in advance of the surgery.

If neither your bed or a hospital bed is an option, you might sleep in a comfortable recliner. For me, I liked being able to change from spending some of the time in my recliner and some in bed. I needed to move around and change my environment a bit to give me the illusion of normal life.

Note: You may wish to purchase a bed rail to help getting in or out of bed.

Choice of Clothes

My recommendation is to wear pull-on, loose-fitting athletic pants with either capris or shorts even in winter. I chose capris. A friend who had knee replacement surgery chose shorts that were a size larger than normal. Shorter pants leave the wound easily accessible to medical personnel—surgeons, nurses, and physical therapists. Athletic clothing makes it easier to dress oneself. I also recommend having several outfits available so can change to clean clothes every day. You might decide not use nightclothes at all and just sleep in the athletic clothing.

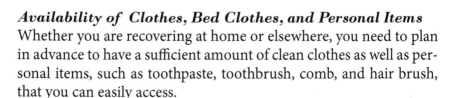

Availability of Clothes, Bed Clothes, and Personal Items

Whether you are recovering at home or elsewhere, you need to plan in advance to have a sufficient amount of clean clothes as well as personal items, such as toothpaste, toothbrush, comb, and hair brush, that you can easily access.

My recovery occurred in my family room, which is on the first floor of my house. I selected clothes, which were kept in the family room, in advance. I kept a change of sheets and blankets nearby as well. My caregiver didn't have to find any of these items because they were in the family room. I wasn't able to change sheets on the bed myself until the end of the second week.

Oops! For a recent surgery. I forgot to put a particular shoe in my family room, where I was living again during recovery. Even though I gave my husband a very specific description of the shoe, he couldn't find it, saying, "All your shoes look alike." That's not true, but to him it was. So I made do with the substitute shoe he found. This is an example of bad planning on my part.

The laundry room in my house is near the family room so I was able to wash clothes, sheets, and blankets as necessary. Admittedly, I didn't wash clothes until the second week, but I had more than enough clean clothes and bed things I had stored in the family room in advance of the surgery.

Follow-up Visits to Surgeon
Make plans for how you're going to get to the surgeon for a follow-up visit. That visit won't be until about 2 weeks after the surgery. At this point the surgeon removes the metal staples. You won't be driving at the time of this follow-up visit. Here was my schedule:

- **June 14:** On this date my surgeon replaced my right knee and "Marie Curie" was born.

- **June 25:** About 2 weeks after the surgery, the surgeon removed the 28 staples. A couple had fallen out before they were removed, which is natural.

- **July 5:** I drove for the first time, which was about 3 weeks after the surgery.

- **July 25:** About 6 weeks after the surgery, the surgeon removed the remaining bandages. I no longer needed to wear a compression sock.

Handicapped Parking Placard

Before the surgery, ask your surgeon to sign a form for a temporary handicapped parking placard from the Department of Motor Vehicles (DMV). Return the signed form to the DMV. Being able to park in handicapped spaces during your recovery is extremely helpful once you're able to drive again. Unless you turn in the signed form in person to the DMV, it may take up to 3 weeks after submitting the form before the placard arrives.

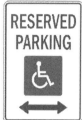

Be Aware: A friend's doctor didn't believe in signing forms for handicapped parking placards for his patients. He felt his patients should walk because it's good exercise even after knee replacement surgery. Frankly, I think the doctor lacked empathy. You only need the placard for just a few weeks.

Set Up Your Home

Stairs

Going up and down stairs is quite helpful. It's the right exercise for recovery. In fact, you can't leave the hospital until the staff shows you how to go up and down stairs. When you're home, just make sure the stairs are cleared of any obstacles and go slowly.

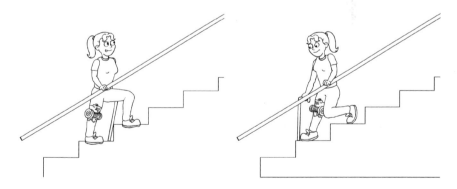

During the first week you won't feel like walking up and down stairs too often because you'll be too tired and won't have much energy. It took me 2 days before I walked up the stairs to the second floor in my house so I could shower. When you walk up or down stairs, do it slowly, one step at a time.

Recommendation: Always use the chair rail. Ideally, two chair rails are best. However, not all stairs include two chair rails so, if possible, use both a cane and chair rail when you're either ascending or descending stairs.

- **Going Up Stairs:** Step up with your good leg first, then step up with your bad leg, i.e., the one with the replaced knee joint, onto the same step.

- **Going Down Stairs:** Step down with your bad leg first, then step down onto the same step with your good leg.

Again, if you live in a second- or third-floor condo or apartment, you need to consider whether that's too many stairs for the first couple of weeks after you're released from the hospital. In fact, you may want to check into a rehabilitation facility or live somewhere else temporarily. Stairs are good exercise, but too many stairs may be far too challenging.

Warning: Remove all throw rugs and anything you can trip on from the floors. You don't want to risk falling on your new knee. If you have pets, watch out for them being under your feet.

Showers and Baths

Advances in medical technology are wonderful. In the 1980s through 2003, I had several foot operations. Taking a shower with a bag on my foot was awkward. I hated it. So, before my knee replacement surgery, I assumed taking showers would become quite a chore once again. Not so. The bandage on the incision allows you to take showers with no problem. I was thrilled beyond words.

Tip: There's nothing as wonderful as taking a shower after surgery as soon as one can. When I take a shower after a surgery, I begin to feel normal even if I'm facing a long recovery.

Surgeons advise against baths and pool therapy for about 6 weeks after surgery. Resume them only if the incision is completely closed and healed. After that time, use a bath seat and a rubber mat or nonskid adhesive strips on the bottom of the bath tub. Your surgeon's office or occupational or physical therapist should give you instructions on how to maneuver into and out of the tub.

Warning: In taking a shower, be careful in stepping over its narrow edge. You don't want to bump into it with the leg on which you've just had surgery. The result is pain.

Bed on the First Floor If Possible

During recovery I spent 6 to 8 weeks on the sofa bed in the family room on my first floor. This was a good idea because it meant I didn't disturb my husband's sleep. Before the surgery, we moved the sofa bed in front of the TV. The worst nerve pain started every night about 11:30 to 1:30 p.m., and it was tremendously disruptive. I would watch TV to distract myself. During the first couple of weeks when I was tired and found it hard to read, write, or use my brain for other worthwhile purposes, watching TV worked well. Having a bed on the first floor where our kitchen, family room, and laundry room are located was ideal for me.

Sleeping on the first floor meant I could reach the refrigerator in the garage, where we kept sodas and the ice for the ice machine. There are four steps to our garage, but I was able to go up and down those steps with care at the end of the first week.

I'm quite independent, but sometimes it's necessary to accept help, such as during recovery from surgery. Setting up your home to have easy access to everything needed, such as bedroom, food, laundry room, and bathroom, lets you be as independent as you want as soon as you can.

Tip: Be smart about when to accept help. It's good to be independent, but it's smart not to push yourself too soon. After all, you want to recover from surgery successfully, not risk damaging yourself.

Comfortable Recliner

After the surgery I didn't want to lie in bed all day. Moving around was good therapy and good for recovery. Lying down all the time puts you at risk for developing blood clots, something you want to avoid at all costs.

Walk, Walk, Walk! Walk every hour after the surgery when you're awake.

Most of the time, I sat in a comfortable leather reclining chair, which allowed me to keep my legs elevated on the separate footstool. If you can, choose either an actual lift-up recliner as shown in the picture or a reclining chair like mine with a separate footstool. You can also use a regular chair and footstool, or you can recline on a sofa, although neither option is as comfortable as a reclining chair or recliner. Make sure the chair, recliner, or sofa has arms that allow you to push yourself up.

My chair was also convenient for using the ice machine, which was positioned between the chair and the sofa bed. From my chair I could read, watch TV, sleep, check email, and so forth.

Note: Make sure to put your legs up. Don't dangle them. I found it very hard to sit in a regular chair in the normal way for several months.

Easy Access to Kitchen and Laundry Room
As I mentioned earlier, sleeping on the first floor allowed me to get into the kitchen and laundry room easily. Since I was up during the night, not having to go up or down stairs to access the kitchen was an important time-saver. I could wash and dry clothes and sheets when needed. Also, because MS and my other diseases cause tremendous fatigue, it was critical not to tire myself unnecessarily.

Important: Even if you're healthy and fit, surgery causes fatigue for the first few weeks due to the effects of anesthesia and the fact your body is recovering. Go with it. Sleep and you'll recover sooner. That being said, however, you'll want to resume a normal schedule as soon as you can.

Easy to Prepare Food

Before the surgery make sure you stock up on food you can easily prepare, particularly if you live by yourself. Buy yogurt, cereals, canned soup, and frozen meals or other items you can quickly prepare with little effort. Don't go crazy in eating sweets and junk food, but a little doesn't matter unless you're diabetic.

Protein at every meal is important for bone healing and provides fuel for the body. Fatigue may occur because your body is not getting enough protein from the food you're eating and is taking it from your muscles, something you want to avoid.

Frozen meals you can microwave or other food that can be prepared quickly may not create the most nutritious diet, but it's practical for the first few weeks of recovery. You may not have someone to make all of your meals.

Tip: A microwave is a good thing to own if you don't already have one.

If you must make your own meals, standing even for short times can be tiring and quite painful. On the other hand, standing for short periods at the sink or microwave is good because bones heal along lines of weight bearing stress.

For me, MS makes standing difficult. Recovery from knee replacement surgery made it impossible. This problem may not affect healthy people recovering from knee replacement surgery as much as it did me, but it may. Be prepared.

Tip: Have a chair in the kitchen in case standing is painful or if you become tired when making a meal.

High-Fiber Diet

Anesthesia and pain medicine can cause constipation. If you haven't had surgery before, you may not think this effect is serious, but it is. It can cause lots of pain. To avoid constipation, keep a high-fiber diet, which means you need fruit and vegetables. If buying fresh fruit and vegetables isn't possible, buy powdered or dry fruits or frozen vegetables in advance.

Consult your primary care physician for recommendations on how to avoid constipation. Be proactive. You don't want to have pain from both your knee and your bowels. Your physician may advise you to start taking either stool softeners or vegetable laxatives as soon as you return home. Then back off taking them as needed. Some popular brands are Colace, Senna, and Miralax.

Important: Due to advice from my gastroenterologist, I not only eat fiber every day but also drink a taste-free fiber supplement. When recovering from surgery, I'm especially careful to do so. Unless your physician says otherwise, it's good advice to follow after surgery.

Children and Pets

Before the surgery, determine who is going to take care of your children and pets. Even if you're a healthy individual, you won't be able to take care of them the day of the surgery, the time you're in the hospital, and for several days, perhaps longer, after you're home.

I own a small dog and two cats. I didn't allow the dog to sit on my lap for a year. The clumsiness of my dog would have been too painful. My cats, who were more graceful and less heavy, did not cause a problem.

Prepare for Boredom!

Surgery and fatigue go hand in hand, but you're not going to sleep all day and your energy levels increase as you recover. Television is an 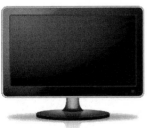 easy fix for boredom during the first week or so you're home because you do sleep a lot. Depending on your reactions to pain medication, your mind probably won't be as alert as it is normally. For example, during the several weeks after surgery, I can't read books. I can read email, which is generally short, on my cell phone or tablet, but books require too much attention and concentration. So during that time I watch TV.

Afterwards, I usually have books and computer games available to me in addition to TV. I write fiction and nonfiction, so I begin writing; but my level of productivity is severely hampered. What are your hobbies, if any? Plan in advance for the things you would enjoy doing during recovery while you're stuck in a chair or bed. It's wonderful when people come to visit you, but those visits don't last all day and you'll get tired.

Facts about Recovery: Over the years I've discovered two facts for me about recovering from any surgery: (1) surgery is a bitch and (2) recovery is boring. I hope this book can help you a tiny bit with the first. For the second, figure out in advance how you can make it less boring. **Some knee replacement patients who are healthy and very energetic don't find recovery boring.** They are able to read, do housework, and catch up on other household tasks. Other healthy patients have similar problems to mine. I hope you're one of the former.

Choose the Right Attire for the Hospital

No one cares how you're dressed at the hospital. If you're in surgery, then you wear the medical gown and ribbed socks they give you, and you're naked under that gown. If you were in a car accident and an ambulance took you to the emergency room (ER), one of the first things they do after making sure you're breathing is take your clothes off. A friend of mine was in a bad car accident in which she had broken ribs. She told me later she was horrified that the nurses in the ER cut off her brand new red suit. Although I sympathized with her, I wasn't surprised. I'd watched enough ER reality shows on television to know what occurs. The reason, of course, is that the ER staff wants to focus on keeping you alive. Clothes prevent them from doing their jobs. Trust me, you want them to do their jobs.

Surgery is the same, although it won't be an emergency. The focus is on you and your life, not on your clothes.

Casual or Athletic Attire

Don't dress up to go to the hospital. Wear very casual clothes, such as athletic attire that is easy to put on and take off. Don't wear tight pants. Your leg is going to be thick with bandages. Bring a robe. I suggest one that opens in front.

Immediately after your surgery you're wheeled to your hospital room. There, when you've recovered somewhat, probably the next day, you can dress yourself. Dressing yourself is initially awkward. After the anesthesia from the surgery wears off, getting dressed can be somewhat painful even if you're taking pain medication.

Flat, Sensible Shoes

Wear flat, sensible shoes to the hospital. They should be easy for you to put on and take off. They shouldn't have shoelaces or other closings, such as Velcro. Bending is very awkward. You won't want to tie shoelaces or mess around with anything else. Also, I wore short socks that were easy to put on and take off.

Wear the same type of shoes during your entire recovery. The shoes should be secure; that is, don't wear shoes that cause you to trip or that fall off your feet easily. Don't wear sandals. The shoes should have backs and provide good support.

Note: You've just had surgery. Don't take risks that may cause further injury.

Jewelry

Leave your wedding rings, watch, earrings, and all other jewelry at home. Jewelry may increase your risk of having any of the following:

- Surgical burns from the use of medical equipment during the operation

- Infection caused by bacteria on the jewelry

- Your circulation being impeded to an extremity

In other words, jewelry can be a threat to your life during a procedure. It's a safety issue.

Other Things to Take to the Hospital

Take your insurance card, any copayment required by your insurance company, a driver's license or photo ID, contact phone numbers, watch, and pocket change.

Get the Right Stuff in Advance of the Surgery

Learn from my mistakes. Even though I researched the surgery, I didn't buy everything I needed before the surgery. I listened to the nurses and the hospital who said things would be offered for me while in the hospital. They were, but I could have saved a lot of money if I bought them on my own in advance. In addition, I had not checked with my insurance company about what my policy covered.

Ask for a Prescription for Nerve Pain

You may or may not experience nerve pain. For my next knee replacement surgery, I plan to ask my primary care physician, not my orthopedic surgeon,[1] for a prescription so I can have it available in advance. Nerve pain is beyond irritating. After my physical therapist told me about medicine for nerve pain, I got a prescription from my primary care physician for gabapentin, one of the medicines that helps relieve nerve pain. The medicine didn't get rid of nerve pain entirely; it simply made it more bearable.

What Is Nerve Pain? Hopefully, it's something you won't experience. For me, it felt like my knee was being repeatedly stabbed. The worst nerve pain occurred in the middle of the night, although sometimes it happened at other times. I found it impossible to sleep until the stabbing pain ended. Nerve pain can also be constant tingling, burning, or prickling. The pain of the surgery is hard, but nerve pain is far worse.

---

1 Not all physicians or surgeons are comfortable in giving you a prescription for nerve pain. All medicines have side effects, and there may be good reason for your physician or surgeon to advise against your taking medicine for nerve pain.

Raised Toilet Seat and/or a Toilet Safety Rail

You'll need a raised toilet seat and/or a stand-alone toilet safety rail. Find out if your insurance company pays for these items. If not, the

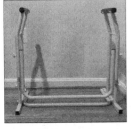 cheapest place to get them is online or a discount store.

I made a mistake and got a raised toilet seat through the hospital after my surgery. My insurance didn't pay for it, and it was expensive to get it through the vendor who supplied it at the hospital. I then ordered a stand-alone toilet safety rail through Amazon because I needed one upstairs as well as the raised toilet seat downstairs.

I found these items quite necessary to get myself up from the toilet for several weeks. Healthier, fit patients may not need to use these items for as long as I did, but they are offered to all people who have knee replacement surgery.

Because of many different surgeries, I keep all the medical paraphernalia I've bought. So I still have both the raised toilet seat and the safety rail. Recently, I used the raised toilet seat during recovery from surgery on my Achilles' tendon. Thank goodness, I kept it! However, if you're in better health than I am, you could always donate or sell the items after your knee replacement surgeries.

Walker

The hospital provided the walker, which was covered by my insurance. However, make sure to check whether your insurance com-

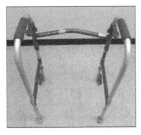 pany covers this item. If not, before the surgery ask the nurse at your surgeon's office or your physical therapist which walker would be best for you to buy. You can buy them online for considerably less than you would pay the hospital. You can also buy them at specialty pharmacy stores or borrow them from organizations that have "medical closets." You can buy padded handle grips for walkers in advance to avoid getting calluses. Some walkers already have them.

Cane

You need to use a cane during recovery from knee replacement surgery. Some hospitals provide canes to patients. If you need to buy a cane, purchase it before your surgery. Depending on your situation—i.e., whether you have complications such as coexisting conditions or diseases—you use the walker for a week or so immediately after the surgery. Then you graduate to using just a cane.

Your physical therapist adjusts the cane for your height and shows you how to use it. Hold the cane in the hand on your "good" side so it provides support to the opposite "bad" side, i.e., the knee on which you've just had surgery.

Advantages of Using Canes: Due to MS, I've used canes for years. Most people don't seem to realize a cane can be a weapon. My canes are made of hard wood. If needed, I could use them to defend myself. A second advantage is using a cane to open elevator doors at the last possible moment without injuring a hand or arm. The look of surprise on the faces of folks in the elevator is more than rewarding. That alone makes me happy, more or less, about needing a cane.

Where to Buy Canes: You can buy inexpensive, adjustable metal canes online or at chain stores, pharmacies, or grocery stores. Sometimes tobacco stores sell canes, although these tend to be more expensive. You might also be able to borrow them from various organizations that have "medical closets."

Ice Machine and Ice

On the advice of a nurse at my surgeon's office, I bought an ice machine before the surgery. Ice machines are expensive. When I bought mine (the picture shows my cat investigating it) in 2014, it was a little over $200. They are available, however, online for less.

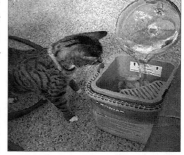

A friend who recently had knee replacement surgery said her hospital rented ice machines to patients for 3

weeks and then patients negotiated for longer use. She used gel packs after the first 3 weeks. Another hospital used gel packs only. My hospital used an ice machine. I used my own ice machine for weeks after returning home.

You'll also need to buy a constant supply of ice. If you live by yourself, make arrangements in advance for someone buy and deliver ice often after you return home. An ice machine uses a lot of ice, more than your refrigerator may be able to supply for an entire day.

Bottom Line: Buy an ice machine. You'll use it often to control the pain and swelling in your leg. It is well worth the price, but the cost is probably not covered by your insurance.

Gel Pack

Since you have osteoarthritis, you may already own and use a gel pack. Gel packs (my frozen one is shown in the picture) are por-

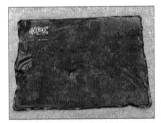 table plastic sacs containing water or a refrigerant gel or liquid that are stored in the freezer until needed. A frozen gel pack absorbs heat, which is needed when you knee is injured through osteoarthritis, after knee replacement surgery, or from other injuries.

Tip: You can use a frozen bag of peas or corn instead of a gel pack. In my experience, however, gel packs work better. Bottom line: Ice machines work best after knee replacement surgery.

In my opinion, gel packs are not nearly as helpful as using an ice machine. Late in your recovery you may prefer to use a gel pack because a gel pack doesn't require ice. That is, it's easier to get the gel pack from the freezer and position it on your knee rather than putting ice into the ice machine and setting it up.

You can purchase gel packs online or at chain stores or pharmacies. If you don't own or can't afford to use a ice machine on your knee, use a gel pack.

Make Your Own Gel Pack: In a recent internet search, I found an interesting article on how to make a gel pack, which you may wish to explore: http://www.spine-health.com/blog/how-make-your-own-gel-ice-pack-or-moist-heat-pack. Another idea is to fill a gallon-size zipped plastic bag with corn syrup and freeze it inside another zipped plastic bag. Place the frozen bag on a towel on your knee. The bag conforms to your knee's shape and stays cold for about 15 minutes.

Vitamin E Gel, Scar Strips, or Cocoa Butter for Scars
Scars can be ugly. No, let me correct that. Scars are definitely ugly. However, some scars are less noticeable than others.

To make scars less noticeable, after the surgeon removes the staples and the bandage from the incision on your knee, use Vitamin E gel, scar strips, or cocoa butter several times a day. These products make the skin moister and less dry and stiff and improve the appearance of the scar. You can find these products online or at grocery stores and pharmacies.

Here are the full names of the products; there may be other brands than those listed available also:

- **Cococare Vitamin E Antioxidant Gel**—Not only do I use this product every day, I use it more frequently after every surgery on scars.

- **ScarAway C-Section Scar Treatment Strips, Silicone Adhesive Soft Fabric 4-Sheets (7 x 1.5 inch)**—Scar strips were designed mostly for women with C-section scars to flatten and fade the scars.

- **Palmer's Cocoa Butter Formula Cream**—My mother swore by cocoa butter for minimizing scars.

A friend who had knee replacement surgery said the fabric scar strips are reusable. She would wear the strips, remove and wash them with mild soap to retain the adhesive, pat them dry, and allow them to air dry, and then reuse them. She wore the strips for about 14 days.

She had to piece more than one strip over the scar because the scar was too long. You can use these strips over both new or old scars to minimize their appearance.

Caveat: If you like scars and feel they provide some oomph to your personality or appearance, disregard this advice. It won't bother me.

Kinesiology Tape

One of the very painful problems I had several times during my recovery was a wandering knee cap, or patella. None of my research warned me about this problem so, when it happened, I wondered if something with the surgery had gone awry.

No, my physical therapist told me. It just happens. She then found the edges of my kneecap and moved it back into place. It was incredibly painful.

The second time my knee cap did a walkabout, I asked the physical therapist to show me how to put it back in place, and she did. Thankfully, I knew how to correct the problem the third and fourth times my kneecap wandered.

The physical therapist then showed me how to use kinesiology tape to keep the kneecap in place; your physical therapist can show you how to apply. You can also review the following videos on YouTube in which they show you how to use the tape to keep your knee stable:

- https://www.youtube.com/watch?v=4gkz4koZVE0

- https://www.youtube.com/watch?v=r4n_XRMY__0

- https://www.youtube.com/watch?v=AAqU0mu3-ic

My Advice: Buy kinesiology tape at your local pharmacy before the surgery so you have it if this problem occurs to you. It's an easy, fairly cheap fix.

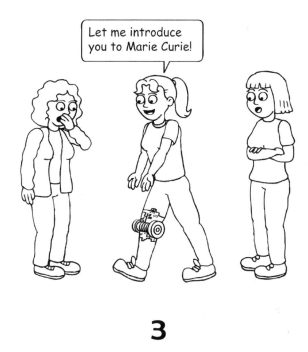

3

Adopt the Right Attitude

Having surgery is not necessarily the end of the world or, more specifically, the end of your life. Yes, surgery can have a bad outcome, but so can driving. It is a risk and one should be aware of the possibilities. However, whining isn't an appealing trait.

Knee replacement surgery is elective surgery. You, the patient, decide that the pain of your osteoarthritic knee is greater than the risk of having the surgery. The payoff is having, eventually, a functional pain-free knee again. Do your homework and be aware of the risk of surgery, but assume the surgery is successful. Don't assume the worst, which guarantees a bad outcome.

Adopt the Right Attitude

After a while—the time varies for each person—the cortisone shots and the exercise you've done to relieve the pain of your arthritic knee no longer work. You've reached the point where replacing the knee becomes your best option. Assuming there are no medical reasons

against having surgery, do it. My mother-in-law was in her late sev-
enties when she had first one knee replaced and then the other 3
months later.

Think positively about the outcome of the surgery. Yes, there may
be pain. My mother-in-law says she had very little pain. Yes, recovery from the surgery involves work on your part. However, the new
knee is worth it. When I'm faced with medical challenges, the phrase
It is what it is comes to mind. These challenges are ones where I
have limited or no more viable options. That is, I have done what I
can do to make whatever it is better and it cannot be made better.
That's the time when you must make a decision and determine how
you can manage the situation. You are facing a challenge—at least,
I found knee replacement surgery quite a challenge. However, I met
that challenge by adopting the right attitude. Say to yourself, "I am a
survivor. It will go well." Never, never, never give up.

Become a Survivor

Being a goal-oriented person, I began telling people a while ago of
my plan to live to 123. When I told a doctor about this, he pooh-
poohed it. He began telling me how horrible it would be to live to
that age. I interrupted him.

"Unless you kill yourself, death comes when death comes," I said.
"I know that living to 123 is unrealistic and old age involves lots of
medical issues. The oldest age to which anyone is known to have
lived is 122—Jeanne Calment of France who died in 1997. I'm com-
petitive, and 123 seemed to be good goal for me. One year better
than Jeanne.

"Look, I write fantasy and science fiction," I said. "Living to 123 is a
great fantasy. It means I have years of living in front of me. In reality, what it really means is that my current medical issue *du jour*
will pass. I will survive. My fantasy bolsters that belief." The doctor
understood and laughed.

My fantasy of living to 123 is part of my telling myself I am lucky. The
more I tell myself of my future ancient age and the more I remind

myself of the different ways in which I am lucky, the more confident I become. It is a survival technique. It's not just one for people like myself who have several medical issues; it's one anyone can adopt. Let me be clear: I'm not suggesting you emulate me by pretending you want to live to an ancient age. My suggestion is always think of yourself as a survivor. If you need surgery, then have it. Do the necessary research, determine if there are any valid serious medical reasons against your having surgery, and do what you need to do to best recover from the surgery. Just don't give up. Remind yourself: Surgery is better than not having it.

Note: The reason I've repeated throughout this book "never, never, never give up" is because when one is ill and in pain— especially if you have chronic lifelong illnesses—one needs to constantly build oneself up psychologically to deal with it.

Get Out of Bed!

After knee replacement surgery, it's important for you to get out of bed and move. There's a risk of deep vein thrombosis (DVT) and pulmonary embolism after the surgery. One of the reasons there's a compression stocking on your leg is to prevent blood clots from forming as well as to minimize swelling.

In the hospital you're given simple physical therapy exercises to do while you're in bed that involve moving your foot. Do them in the hospital and at home! When you return home, make sure you get out of bed often. Force yourself to do for yourself as soon as you can.

Important: A recent study reported that pulmonary embolism is one of the most frequent causes of mortality following total hip and knee replacements.

Practice Saying "Exciting!"

Physical therapy provided lots of challenges to me. Although my range of motion both before and after the surgery was quite good, the exercises often hurt. After all, one has a 6¼-inch incision down the middle of one's leg! Yet I saw great benefits from doing the exercises. When the physical therapist came up with another challenging exercise for me to try, my response was "Exciting!" Of course, saying "exciting" didn't mean I was happy about the prospect. Some of the exercises were more than I wanted to try, although I believe I did all of them. Some were quite difficult at the beginning, but I saw progress over time.

Because of my diseases and the nerve pain, my recovery time was twice as long as healthy people. It amazed me to know people who were able to spend just 3 months or less in physical therapy and then have surgery on the second knee. I must admit I was somewhat envious, but it is what it is. Saying "Exciting!" allowed me to focus on what I needed to do and not be depressed about the time it took for my recovery. The bottom line is that, after 6 months of physical therapy, my knee began to feel much better. After a year, it felt fine. Whether you're healthy or if you've got complications, concentrate on beating my record for recovery! In any event, think positive. It helps.

Create an Imaginary Dartboard

I sometimes worked with irritating people during my career, something to which we can all relate. Since I couldn't show my real feelings and don't approve of violence, I would imagine a dartboard

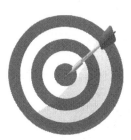

whose target featured a photograph of a problematic individual. Then I would imagine throwing darts at the dartboard. Naturally, my darts always hit the center of the target, which was quite satisfying. As I matured, I began to put whatever, not *whomever,* was bugging me in the center of the dartboard. Again, I threw imaginary darts.

During the knee saga, my right knee occupied the target for quite a while, both before and definitely after the surgery. Hitting the target did not relieve the pain, but it gave me the illusion of doing something about it. The imaginary dartboard helped motivate me to either prepare for or recover from the surgery. If you're not as imaginative or goal oriented as I am, the imaginary dartboard may not prove helpful to you. However, if your personality shares similarities with mine, creating and using an imaginary dartboard is just another device to keep you focused on what needs to be done: recovery with good grace. I find the idea of an imaginary dartboard amusing.

Name Your Knee!

Several months before my surgery, it occurred to me my leg would soon house an artificial implant, i.e., that I would be a cyborg). Therefore, surgery would be the birth of my new artificial knee and the knee would need a name. The idea of naming my new knee amused me. I could swear at my new knee by calling it by name.

Since I'm female, the name would ideally be female. I didn't want to give my knee just any old name. It needed to mean something. What name would I choose?

Note: If you find the idea of naming your new knee and issuing a birth certificate idiotic, don't. We just have a totally different sense of humor.

Because I admire women scientists, the name came to me in a flash: Marie Curie. She was the first female scientist whose biography I had read and who impressed me. Somehow naming my knee *Marie Curie* seemed the right thing to do. I'm not sure she would approve of the

idea, but perhaps, wher-ever she is, she finds it as humorous as I do. After all, I truly do admire her.

My advice to you is to name your new knee. If both of your knees must be replaced, con-

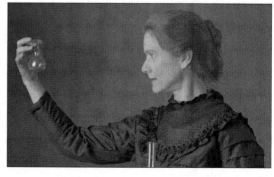

sider a theme. Mine is female scientists. I haven't decided on the scientist I'll choose for my left knee yet. It is, after all, an important decision. If a female scientist comes up with a cure for MS before my left knee needs replacement, then the name of that scientist has first dibs.

Issue a Birth Announcement for Your New Knee

Before my surgery I wrote the birth announcement for Marie Curie, which I sent to myself in an email message. After the surgery when I was in my hospital room and had access to my cell phone, I put a picture of me on the hospital bed and the birth announcement on Facebook for my friends.

After the birth announcement, my friends would ask during my recovery, "How's Marie Curie?" Laughter often accompanied our conversations, even if I complained about Marie being a bitch, because talking about one's knee in the third person is amusing.

> ### Birth Announcement
> Alexis and Chuck Dupree (especially Alexis) are pleased
> to announce the birth of Marie Curie Dupree, Alexis'
> right knee replacement.
> "Thank God for Marie Curie!" Alexis said. "It's been a
> long metaphorical pregnancy to reach the point of birth. We
> are now settling down to the physical accommodation phase
> of knee infancy. There's no cooing, cuddling, or cute baby
> clothes, just physical therapy and lots of ice while we get
> used to each other."
> The Goddess, Alexis' alter ego, will help Alexis during
> the first weeks or months of infancy. Chuck's mom,
> Marcelle Dupree, is also coming to assist. She is, after all,
> the proud grandmother of Marie Curie. No doubt her own
> relatively new knees will welcome Marie into the trending
> knee replacement community.
> Born: June 10, 2014, around 9:30 a.m.
> Where: Circa Hospital, Nearme, Mystate

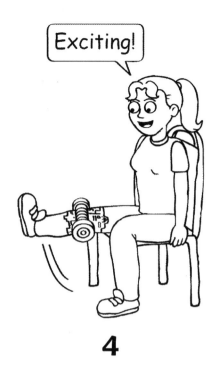

4

Do the Right Thing

If you're someone who likes to take risks or doesn't want to do the right thing, consider abandoning those traits when you're recovering from surgery. You can always resume your normal ways after recovery. Let me explain: Surgery and taking unnecessary risks don't mix well together. There are consequences. Bottom line: It often means more pain and longer recovery.

True Story: One of my coworkers had his knee replaced about 2 years before I had my surgery. He ignored medical advice, didn't do the physical therapy exercises, and returned to work too soon. Admirable, right? Well, no, not really. He damaged his knee so badly he had to have the surgery again! He was a smart man, but he wasn't medically savvy.

My co-worker's story makes me cringe. I'm not looking forward to having my second knee replacement surgery whenever my left knee decides to become more cantankerous than it is now. When the cartilage on that knee gives up the ghost, I'll schedule the surgery. I won't be happy about it, but, having gone through surgery on my right knee, I know what to do to make it successful.

Learn Some Quick Facts about Recovery

Here are some quick facts:

- **Sitting at a desk is hard for a while.** How long "for a while" is depends on the individual. If you're healthy, it may be only 2 to 3 months. I began sitting at my desk in 4 months for short periods of time, 1 to 2 hours. It took me a year to feel comfortable—by that I mean pain free—sitting all day at my desk.

- **Riding as a passenger in a car for over 45 minutes may present issues during the first months of recovery.** I took a 3-hour trip with my husband. It caused major, painful muscle problems that lasted for months.

- **Driving too soon for longer than 40 minutes can also be problematic.** In other words, it may cause fatigue and make your new knee hate you; i.e., pain.

- **Nerve pain may continue for months for some people.** I find nerve pain the worst type of pain, but not everyone has it.

- **Learn to say "no."** Don't overcommit yourself in the first few months of recovery. Once you're driving, going to physical therapy a couple times a week, and beginning to resume normal life, you may not realize that the surgery is still affecting your energy level. Example: A few months after her knee was replaced, a friend tried to resume her former pace of activities. Her fatigue and the pain in her knee were overwhelming. Because her recovery was going well, she had overestimated what she could realistically accomplish.

Don't Overcommit Too Soon. Full recovery takes up to a year for most people. Be push yourself to do too much too soon. If you do, you may pay the price in pain and fatigue. It's very annoying.

Physical Therapy Is Your Friend

Physical therapy begins in the hospital. First, you're instructed to move your foot on the affected leg several times an hour. Then on the second day you learn the correct procedure for walking up and down stairs and for sitting and getting out of a car. Those are skills you need going home.

Depending on your surgeon, a physical therapist comes to your house either the first day or up to 2 weeks after the surgery 2 or 3 times a week. You perform a few simple exercises, which at the time aren't easy. They hurt. You may go outside to walk a short way. The purpose of the exercises is to restore a normal range of motion.

You can begin driving in about 3 to 6 weeks after you leave the hospital. In about 6 to 8 weeks you drive to a physical therapy facility and experience the full joy of an hour of exercises. You'll have physical therapy for 2 or 3 months. I had it for 6 months because of my coexisting illnesses.

Physical therapy can be a pain, literally. However, take it seriously. It works, although you may not see immediate results. You need to be patient—boring, I know. Constant repetition of the exercises helps.

Note: Surgery is an assault on your body, and you need to help your body recover. Recovery from knee replacement surgery takes time, patience, and constant focus on doing what you need to do; i.e., the physical therapy exercises.

As someone with chronic diseases, I've learned that managing them is a full-time job, not one I wanted but one fate assigned me. *C'est le vie.* Recovering from surgery is also a job, although only a temporary one. Like me, you probably don't want it, but you're stuck with it.

Important: Treat recovery as a job. You can either do it well or as well as you're able to, or you can whine and do it halfheartedly and get results you're not happy with. You choose.

I'm a very imaginative, although practical, person. To make things like physical therapy, which to me is boring to the max, more interesting, I tried to think of it as training for a game. The game, of course, was being able to walk again normally without pain. I wanted to win at that game, so I tried my best—I did the physical therapy exercises religiously—and I won. It took me twice as long as most folks, but what a joy it was to hear the surgeon say 3 months postsurgery that my walk looked perfect. It took 6 months of physical therapy to be able to walk up and down stairs in the normal way and a year to be able to sit comfortably at my desk. Pain continued, although lessened each month, for a year. On the anniversary of the surgery, the pain from my replaced knee had disappeared.

For faster and better recovery, pay attention to doing the physical therapy exercises.

Control Pain and Swelling

After surgery, your knee and leg swell—a lot. Swelling is the body's natural reaction and is quite painful. The swelling stays for weeks. In my case, it stayed for months because my body apparently has a love affair with inflammation. If you're healthy, your body probably acts much more reasonably.

In addition, the bruising on your leg make it look like it was run over by a Mack truck. You'll be amazed at how horrible the bruising is. I was. At the time of my knee replacement surgery, earlier surgeries included four previous foot surgeries and an ankle surgery. All of those surgeries had bruising, but nothing as bad as with the knee surgery. However, the bruising eventually disappears.

So here is what I did during recovery from the surgery:

- Iced my knee

- Took pain medication

- Controlled nerve pain by taking gabapentin and by wrapping my knee in cellophane (described later)

- Got frequent massages

- Got trigger point injections of all-natural ingredients

- Used Jaxsens cream often

Tip for Preventing Swelling: Elevate your leg above the level of your heart four to five times daily to help prevent swelling. To elevate your leg, place it on three or four pillows or on a folded-over body pillow.

Ice Your Knee

I used my ice machine to ice my knee several times a day. Be careful, because using it more than 20 minutes at a time may cause frostbite, which is serious.

True Story: Someone I know had toe surgery, used ice too long, and developed frostbite. She didn't use an ice machine, but ice is ice no matter how you apply it. Don't emulate her! Don't use the ice machine for longer than recommended.

As I mentioned in chapter 2, you can also use a gel pack. Frankly, in my opinion, gel packs don't cut it for providing enough relief in the first few weeks after knee surgery. On the other hand, they *do* help.

The Problem with Ice Machines: They fail after a period of time. I planned to use the ice machine I had purchased for the knee replacement surgery for another surgery 2 years later. It worked for 2 days, then the seal around the lid failed. The manufacturer wouldn't repair the machine and replacements parts were no longer available. Obviously, this is a strategy to make clients buy a new machine. All this being said, I do not regret buying the machine in the first place. It was well worth purchasing the ice machine for the knee replacement surgery. If you can afford it, buy it. Some hospitals rent the machines.

Take the Pain Medications

Use the pain medications the surgeon's office prescribed for you, making sure you take them on time and with or without food according to the instructions. Missing a scheduled dose means you won't get the pain relief as soon as you need it. Also, take the medicine exactly as prescribed; i.e., never take more than prescribed. There may be serious side effects.

Control Nerve Pain If You Have It

Many people, but not all, who have knee replacement surgery or any joint replacement surgery experience nerve pain. It drove me crazy. After I returned home from the hospital, the nerve pain would usually begin at night and didn't stop for at least an hour. My leg and knee experienced sharp, shooting, and stabbing pains one after another. It would wake me if I had fallen asleep, and I wouldn't be able to fall back to sleep until it stopped. None of the pain medications helped.

In desperation one night, I searched through YouTube, an invaluable resource, and watched a video by a man who had two knee replacement surgeries. He applied cream on his knee and leg and then wrapped it tightly in cellophane. In essence, he made a poultice. I tried his procedure and it helped me a lot. At physical therapy I described the procedure to another knee replacement patient who complained about nerve pain. She tried it and liked it as well.

Cellophane Poultice for Nerve Pain: Here's the YouTube link: http://www.youtube.com/watch?v=bt1eTx3k9ns

---

The physical therapists told me about gabapentin, a medicine prescribed to help relieve nerve pain. Like many medicines, it is used for other problems. Ask for a prescription for nerve pain from your primary care physician or neurologist if you have one. Not all orthopedic surgeons are comfortable in prescribing such medicine.

Get a Massage

If you can afford it—insurance probably won't pay for it, get a medical massage of the affected leg and your whole body after you're able to drive. I'm not talking about a massage at a salon—usually, those massage therapists don't do medical massages; i.e., I haven't found any to be knowledgeable enough. Sometimes physical therapists can do some limited massage as part of physical therapy or they know of massage therapists.

The chiropractors I see on a regular basis have a massage therapist who I saw twice a week for 6 months. I realize this is not an option for most people, but for people who have MS and fibromyalgia, it's very important. If you can't afford to have frequent massages, try to get at least one.

Do Your Own Massage: You can also massage your own leg by stroking it from the mid-calf toward the hip to help move fluid and desensitize numb or painful areas.

Massages are quite effective in getting rid of swelling. Following my first massage after the surgery, the physical therapist who I saw later that day noted that the swelling in my leg had decreased by 3 cm. That's an incredible reduction.

Get Trigger Point Injections of All-Natural Ingredients

I see my chiropractors once or twice a week for trigger point injections, usually into my lower back for fibromyalgia. The ingredients of the trigger point injections are mostly anti-inflammatory herbs, although they also contain a very small amount of Lidocaine and Ketolorac. My insurance covers the injections.

The only reason I get trigger point injections is because they work. After my knee replacement surgery, I had injections below my knee to reduce the pain.

Either a physician or a nurse must give the injections. If you want to explore this option, ask your physician to call my chiropractors' office, which is Ashburn Pain Management and Wellness Center, 20955 Professional Plaza, Suite 320, Ashburn, Virginia 20147. The phone number is 571-918-0795. The chiropractors are Dr. Mike and Tara Urschel. Dr. Kraig D. Moore gives the injections.

Use Jaxsens Cream

During my recovery I used Jaxsens cream, an herbal pain relief cream that was created by Dr. Moore and Drs. Urschel of the Ashburn Pain Management and Wellness Center. Jaxsens cream, which contains mostly anti-inflammatory herbal ingredients, must be applied 3 or 4 times a day to the area of your body in pain. It works better the more you use it, which is a characteristic of herbal creams. You may not feel tremendous relief the first time you apply it, but the cumulative effect is powerful. I think it works far better than any other pain cream available.

True Story: Recently, I traveled to New Zealand where I stayed with a woman who had terrible back pain. Although she had seen doctors and undergone several tests, no one had been able to diagnose the problem. I gave her a tube of Jaxsens and told her how to use it. Three weeks after I returned home, she sent me a text telling me as long as she used the Jaxsens her pain was gone. She now receives a steady supply of Jaxsens.

I get Jaxsens directly from the chiropractors who I see weekly. It's also available through Wegmans grocery store. The Urschels plan to make it available through other venues. To find out more about Jaxsens and how to get the product, go to the Jaxsens website: http://www.jaxsens.com.

Try K-Laser Therapy If Available
I'm currently in physical therapy for issues unrelated to my right knee replacement. Another patient, who had just undergone knee replacement surgery, told me he received laser therapy to deal with the pain and inflammation. I've now received several laser treatments on my current problems. The pain and inflammation have decreased significantly; the scars from recent surgeries are much reduced in size. The treatment is pain free and doesn't involve drugs, needles, or surgery.

This treatment is not available everywhere. However, you can search for providers in your area on the K-Laser therapy website: https://www.k-laser.com/.

Recommendation: When my left knee is replaced, I plan to use K-Laser therapy as soon as possible after the surgery.

Do as Much for Yourself as Soon as You Can
My advice for recovering from any surgery is to be as self-reliant as possible as soon as it's reasonable. When you first return home,

sleeping and resting form a majority of your day. You won't feel like doing much. The anesthesia makes you tired for about a week or so after the surgery.

When I came home, I wanted to take a shower, something I was unable to do in the hospital. So the second day home I went upstairs slowly one step at a time to my master bathroom and showered. What a relief it was to feel clean! Then I made the slow trip downstairs. By the time I was downstairs, I collapsed in our sofa bed and took a nap.

Advice: As you become more alert, do as much for yourself as soon as you can. Listen to your body. Don't do too much. You'll know when you've done too much—pain increases and you'll need to sleep. Sleep is very important for recovering from surgery.

During the first 2 weeks after I came home, I iced my knee, took a shower, watched television, talked to my mother-in-law, and slept. Even though I like to read, my mind was too affected by the anesthesia and the prescription medicine to be able to concentrate well enough to read for long.

Deal with Any Complications Immediately

Contact your surgeon if you have a complication. Only call if there's a legitimate concern.

Prescriptions
On the first day home, one of the prescribed medications made me throw up. So I called my surgeon's office immediately and got a different prescription, which my husband picked up at the pharmacy.

Blood Clot
I also had major widespread bruising, which was more than I had experienced with previous surgeries. Because I was concerned about the possibility of a blood clot, I called the surgeon's office. Fortunately, the bruising turned out to be normal, but I was glad I called.

Understand Surgery Details (Frequently Asked Questions)

This section answers a few frequently asked questions.

How Long Are You in the Hospital?

I was in the hospital for a little over 2 days. I showed up early one morning and had the surgery. In the hospital where the surgery was performed, all patients who were having joint replacement surgery were in the same ward. Patients had their own rooms, to avoid the possibility of infection.

Note: The number of days in the hospital depends on the hospital. Some hospitals keep people for less time. Whether you have a private room also depends on the hospital.

When Can You Walk Again after Surgery?

Much, much quicker than you would think possible. After you have the surgery and are being wheeled on the gurney from the recovery room to your hospital room, the aides stop the gurney outside your room. They give you a walker and require you to walk from the gurney to the bed in your hospital room. That sounds awful, doesn't it? It isn't. Your leg is still anesthetized so you don't feel pain. Walking to the bed is just a bit awkward.

Can You Take Electronic Devices to the Hospital?

I didn't have any problems in doing so. Of course, I took only my cell phone to the hospital; nothing else. I have a cell phone case, which I wear most of the time, that hangs around my neck, making the cell phone fairly secure. I gave it to my husband while I was in surgery. However, the hospital suggested that patients leave electrical items at home. Ask the nurses at your surgeon's office for their advice.

Will Hospital Employees Steal Your Possessions?

I suppose it could happen. I've never had any problems with any of my surgeries. Then again, the only possessions I took with me were my clothes, shoes, personal hygiene items, watch, and my cell phone. I also took my insurance card and driver's license, which I gave to my husband after hospital registration.

Can I Bring Books or Crafts, Like Sewing or Knitting to the Hospital?

Sure, but you won't feel much like doing anything except sleeping or dozing. I tried to watch TV and I did play simple computer games on my cell phone, but not for long. When I'm in the hospital, I'm rarely awake. Also, I don't have the ability to focus much on anything. Pain drugs make me fairly stupid. The anesthesia from the surgery makes you tired for about a week. Nurses wake you in the middle of the night to take your vitals, which is important, and give you medicine, which you want. So you're just tired.

True Story: Many years ago major surgery put me in the hospital for a week. I took several books. The pain, the stupidity I felt from the pain medication, and fatigue prevented me from opening a single one.

What Kind of Knee Replacement Hardware Will You Receive?

My surgeon's office gave patients a book about knee replacement surgery that explained which replacement hardware they used. I went with the best surgeon I could find and trusted his choice of hardware. That seemed better to me at the time than insisting on a particular piece of hardware, especially since I'm not a medical professional.

Is Your Knee in a Cast? Does It Have Stitches?

For my knee surgery I had staples closing the incision. The staples were removed in about 2 weeks. The staples were covered with a thin see-through bandage, which eventually falls off. My leg was bandaged and I wore a compression stocking. The bandages were removed and the compression stocking was no longer needed after about 6 weeks.

When Can You Drive?

The time varies for each person and on which leg the surgery is performed. On average, patients begin driving about 3 to 4 weeks after leaving the hospital. Some people can drive as early as 2 weeks; some can't drive until 6 weeks.

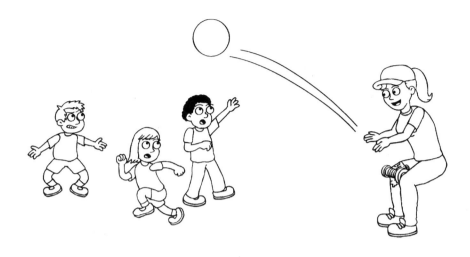

5

Live with Your New Knee

Once you've fully recovered from surgery, your new knee is a miracle. When I go to the pool now and stand only on my right leg, which is one of the physical therapy exercises I did before and after the surgery, the knee is as sturdy as a rock.

Mobility

It takes about a year to fully recover from knee replacement surgery even if you're a healthy person. That doesn't mean you won't be able to do things long before the year is up. It means that after a year you won't have any limitations. During that year of recovery, depending on your health before the surgery, you may find that your recovery is much better and sooner than others. Most people take about 3 months or less to be able to resume most activities. It was 6 months for me and then I continued to have limitations on some activities. However, even though I had pain and had difficulties going up and down stairs in the normal way, 6 months after the surgery I went to Madrid and Segovia with my husband. I walked a lot. Although I limited myself to one or two major activities a day, I pushed myself. However, I sat down when I needed to do so. I took portable ice packs with me to put on my knee after I got back to the hotel and took a 2-hour nap each day. It was a wonderful trip because I managed the knee pain along with my daily MS symptoms.

Note: If you're a healthy person, you'll probably do quite well 3 months after the surgery, although you may experience some pain and more fatigue than usual. However, your surgeon may be reluctant to approve of out of the country travel until 4 months postsurgery.

Kneeling the first 6 months to a year may be interesting; that is, awkward or painful. Everything depends on how active you are or have been until now. Because I exercised the year before my surgery, my range of motion was quite good, but kneeling was painful. Now it's slightly awkward, not painful.

Physical Therapy for Kneeling: A friend who had knee replacement surgery said her physical therapist added an exercise to her routine for kneeling. My physical therapy didn't include that exercise, so I'm doing it now. Ask your physical therapist to show you the exercise.

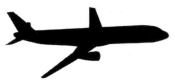

Travel with Your New Knee

Now that you have a new knee, you can look forward to setting off the security monitors at airports.

Tell Security about Your Knee Replacement

As mentioned, your new knee replacement sets off monitors at airports. Tell security immediately, "I have a knee replacement." They'll whisk you off to the monitor where you need to hold your hands above your head. The knee still sets off the monitor. It's very exciting. Not. On the other hand, I've found it quicker to get through security than going through the other monitors, especially when it's crowded.

Apply to TSA Pre

To get through security in the United States more quickly, it's a good idea to apply to TSA Pre. I like it because I don't have to wait in long lines and I don't have to take my shoes off. A friend whose husband had knee replacement surgery earlier suggested my applying, and I've been pleased ever since.

Be Aware: There is a charge for TSA Pre. You need to apply for it, then let TSA take fingerprints and investigate you. There is a waiting period before you are approved.

Fly Business Class If Possible While in Recovery

When I met my husband in Spain 6 months after my surgery, I flew business class. The only reason I was able to do so was because my husband travels overseas often and had many frequent flyer miles, which he used for my tickets. At that time I would not have been able to fly coach because of the knee pain.

Note: At 6 months following knee replacement surgery, flying coach shouldn't be a problem for healthy people.

Flying business class is not an option for everyone, nor is it necessary for everyone who has had knee replacement surgery. Again, it depends on you. If you're healthy, flying coach may not be a problem.

Ask for a Wheelchair While in Recovery

If your knee hasn't totally healed, ask for a wheelchair at airports. This advice is practical. If you're traveling and need to walk the long routes some airports force you to take to get to the gate or baggage claim, ask for a wheelchair when you purchase your tickets. If it's not necessary—i.e., you're not going to have tremendous fatigue or pain, then walk. When I traveled to Spain, I had a wheelchair at every airport. I only request wheelchairs if I need them.

Don't overestimate your energy, a problem healthy people who've had surgery often do. If in doubt, take a wheelchair.

Note: The best advice is don't take a trip too early in your recovery from knee replacement surgery if you can avoid it.

Use Ice Packs While in Recovery Overseas

Years ago I discovered that European hotels lack ice machines. Hotels in New Zealand don't have them either. Because I had traveled to Europe several times prior to my trip to Spain, I packed lots of ice packs to use on my knee. I limited the amount of walking I did in Spain. However, I used every single ice pack while I was there to help relieve the pain in my knee.

Ice Packs to the Rescue: Outside the United States, many hotels, perhaps all, don't have ice machines. So pack ice packs on overseas visits if you're still having knee pain. You can buy ice packs online or at pharmacies or other stores. A friend who traveled overseas after her surgery asked the bar at the hotel where she stayed for ice, which is another alternative.

Use an Antibiotic before Dental Appointments

Some surgeons, not all, ask you to make a practice of taking an antibiotic an hour before any dental appointment, including cleanings. The purpose behind this advice is to avoid any possible infection that may occur in your artificial joint. Get the prescription from your primary care physician.

Should You Really Take the Antibiotic? Yes, I think so, but I'm not a physician so check with your surgeon. Personally, I don't want to have any more illness than I already have in my life. An infection in my knee joint might mean more surgery or some other procedure on the knee. I want to avoid that like the plague. Everyone, however, is entitled to make his or her own decision. If you like to gamble, so be it.

Resume Normal Life

Life after full recovery from knee replacement surgery goes back to normal. Your knee functions well, and you don't notice any difference from your memories of your own knee when it worked as it should. Well, of course, it does set off security monitors. This change is small in the greater scheme of things. The main point is that your knee no longer causes excruciating pain!

One caveat: Artificial knee joints last about 20 years, possibly longer. In all honesty, I don't look forward to the possibility of having my right knee replaced if it fails after 20 years. Knowing that my left knee may lose its battle with osteoarthritis at some point in time doesn't make me happy either. That being said, I'm positive I'll be able to deal with those surgeries when they occur. I'm a survivor. I recover from surgeries well because I work at doing so.

Last Word of Advice: Surgery is a bitch and recovery is boring (at least to me), but you can get through it. May you triumph over your surgery and recovery!

Would You Please?

If you've received any value from this book, I'd like to ask you for a favor. Would you be kind enough to leave a review for this book on Amazon, Goodreads, Barnes & Noble, iTunes, and other review sites? Thank you.

A

Checklists

This appendix includes the following sections, which were described in Chapter 2, in a format that leaves room for notes and comments:

- <u>"Orthopedic Surgeons" on page 56</u>—Record the information about orthopedic surgeons you're considering in this section.

- <u>"Insurance Information" on page 60</u>—Find out what your medical insurance policy covers and record the answers here.

- <u>"Rehabilitation Centers" on page 64</u>—List information about rehabilitation centers, if needed, in this section.

- <u>"Physical Therapy Centers" on page 68</u>—Record information about physical therapy centers on these pages.

- <u>"Preparation for Surgery" on page 72</u>—Review the things to do or acquire that are listed in this checklist before the surgery.

- <u>"Birth Announcement" on page 74</u>—Write, if you wish, a birth announcement for your new artificial knee.

Orthopedic Surgeons

Surgeon _____

_____

Web Site _____

Address _____

_____

City _____

State _____ Zip _____

Phone _____

Fax _____

Recommended by _____

_____

_____

Comments _____

_____

_____

_____

_____

_____

_____

_____

_____

_____

_____

_____

_____

_____

Orthopedic Surgeons

Surgeon _____

_____

Web Site _____

Address _____

City _____

State _____ Zip _____

Phone _____

Fax _____

Recommended by _____

_____

_____

Comments _____

_____

_____

_____

_____

_____

_____

_____

_____

_____

_____

_____

Surgeons

Orthopedic Surgeons

Surgeon

Web Site
Address

City
State   Zip
Phone
Fax
Recommended by

Comments

Orthopedic Surgeons

Surgeon _____

_____

_____

Web Site _____

Address _____

_____

City _____

State _____ Zip _____

Phone _____

Fax _____

Recommended by _____

_____

_____

_____

Comments _____

_____

_____

_____

_____

_____

_____

_____

_____

_____

_____

_____

_____

_____

_____

Surgeons

Insurance Information

Does your policy cover the following:

The surgery, including cost of surgeon, anesthesiologist, hospital, etc.?

☐ Yes

☐ No

Limitations and copay? _____

_____

A walker?

☐ Yes

☐ No

Limitations and copay? _____

A cane?

☐ Yes

☐ No

Limitations and copay? _____

A raised toilet seat or toilet safety rail?

☐ Yes

☐ No

Limitations and copay? _____

Ice machine?

☐ Yes

☐ No

Limitations and copay? _____

Insurance

Insurance Information

Hospital bed (if needed)?

☐ Yes

☐ No

Limitations and copay? _____

Rehabilitation centers (if needed)?

☐ Yes

☐ No

Limitations and copay? _____

Insurance

Physical therapy?

☐ Yes

☐ No

Limitations and copay? _____

Additional comments (record more notes on following pages):

_____

_____

_____

_____

_____

_____

_____

_____

_____

_____

_____

_____

_____

Insurance Information

Record information about your medical insurance policy here.

_____

_____

_____

_____

_____

_____

_____

_____

_____

_____

_____

_____

_____

_____

_____

_____

_____

_____

_____

_____

_____

_____

_____

_____

Insurance

Insurance Information

Record information about your medical insurance policy here.

_____

_____

_____

_____

_____

_____

_____

_____

_____

Insurance

_____

_____

_____

_____

_____

_____

_____

_____

_____

_____

_____

_____

_____

_____

_____

_____

Rehabilitation Centers

Rehabilitation Center _____

Contact _____

Web Site _____
Address _____

City _____
State _____ Zip _____
Phone _____
Fax _____
Comments _____

Contact Information for Integral Team Members at Center

_____
_____
_____
_____
_____
_____
_____
_____
_____
_____
_____
_____
_____
_____

Rehabilitation

Rehabilitation Centers

Rehabilitation Center _____

Contact _____

Web Site _____
Address _____

City _____
State _____ Zip _____
Phone _____
Fax _____
Comments _____

_____

Contact Information for Integral Team Members at Center

_____
_____
_____
_____
_____
_____
_____
_____
_____
_____
_____
_____
_____
_____
_____

Rehabilitation

Rehabilitation Centers

Rehabilitation Center _____

Contact _____

Web Site _____
Address _____

City _____
State _____ Zip _____
Phone _____
Fax _____
Comments _____

Contact Information for Integral Team Members at Center

_____
_____
_____
_____
_____
_____
_____
_____
_____
_____
_____
_____
_____

Rehabilitation

Rehabilitation Centers

Rehabilitation Center _____

Contact _____

Web Site
Address _____

City _____
State _____ Zip _____
Phone _____
Fax _____
Comments _____

_____

Contact Information for Integral Team Members at Center

_____
_____
_____
_____
_____
_____
_____
_____
_____
_____
_____
_____
_____
_____
_____

Rehabilitation

Physical Therapy Centers

Physical Therapy Center _____

Contact _____

Web Site _____
Address _____

City _____
State _____ Zip _____
Phone _____
Fax _____
Comments _____

_____
_____
_____
_____
_____

PT

_____
_____
_____
_____
_____
_____
_____
_____
_____
_____

Physical Therapy Centers

Physical Therapy Center _____

Contact _____

Web Site _____
Address _____

City _____
State _____ Zip _____
Phone _____
Fax _____
Comments _____

_____
_____
_____
_____
_____
_____
_____
_____
_____
_____
_____
_____
_____
_____
_____
_____
_____

PT

Physical Therapy Centers

Physical Therapy Center _____

_____

Contact _____

_____

Web Site _____

Address _____

_____

City _____

State _____ Zip _____

Phone _____

Fax _____

Comments _____

_____

_____

_____

_____

_____

_____

_____

_____

_____

_____

_____

_____

_____

_____

_____

_____

Physical Therapy Centers

Physical Therapy Center _____

Contact _____

Web Site _____

Address _____

City _____

State _____ Zip _____

Phone _____

Fax _____

Comments _____

PT

Preparation for Surgery

SET THINGS UP IN ADVANCE AND SET UP YOUR HOME

Even if you're going to a rehabilitation center, you should do the
following things so that your home is set up for your return.
Make sure the following items are available near where you're
sleeping so that you can access them easily:

- ☐ Do you have a bed of normal height on the first floor?
- ☐ Did you arrange for a hospital bed if needed?
- ☐ Two or three sets of casual clothes, socks, and a pair of flat sensible shoes.
- ☐ An extra set of bed clothes; i.e., sheets and blankets.
- ☐ Personal items, such as toothpaste, toothbrush, soap, hairbrush, comb, etc., in a nearby bathroom.
- ☐ Do you have a comfortable recliner or substitute such as a chair and footstool?
- ☐ Is your bed near the kitchen and laundry room?
- ☐ If the bed is a sofa bed, make sure it's set up and bed clothes are on it before you leave for surgery.
- ☐ Is your bed near a powder room or bathroom?
- ☐ Do you have someone to drive you to the surgeon's office for a follow-up visit?
- ☐ Have you moved throw rugs and other items in your pathway that might trip you?
- ☐ Do you have easy to prepare food, fruit, and vegetables?
- ☐ Do you a way to replenish food when you run out? In other words, is there someone who can get groceries for you if needed?
- ☐ Do you have at least a monthly supply of a fiber supplement to help deal with constipation?
- ☐ Do you have a microwave oven?
- ☐ Is someone going to take care of your children and/or your pets during your recovery?
- ☐ Do you have enough books, movies, or other items to help you fight boredom?

Checklist

Preparation for Surgery

- ☐ Is your bed and recliner set up to watch TV easily?
- ☐ Do you have a handicapped parking placard?

CHOOSE THE RIGHT ATTIRE FOR THE HOSPITAL

- ☐ Wear casual or athletic attire.
- ☐ Wear flat sensible shoes.
- ☐ Leave all jewelry (include wedding and engagement rings) at home.

GET THE RIGHT STUFF IN ADVANCE OF THE SURGERY

- ☐ Ask for a prescription for nerve pain from your primary care physician.
- ☐ Do you have a seat for your bathtub (unless you're using a shower)?
- ☐ Do you have a raised toilet seat and/or a toilet safety rail?
- ☐ Do you have a walker?
- ☐ Do you have a cane?
- ☐ Do you have an ice machine?
- ☐ Do you have ice and a way to replenish or buy ice after it's used?
- ☐ Do you have a gel pack?
- ☐ Do you have Vitamin E gel, scar strips, or cocoa butter?
- ☐ Do you have kinesiology tape?

Checklist

Birth Announcement

You may find it just as amusing as I to name your new artificial joint. Think of the possibilities of swearing at it or simply referring to it as a member of your family, which in a way it is.

Remember: If you think naming your new knee or issuing a birth announcement is idiotic, don't.

Here's the birth announcement I issued on Facebook for you to use as an example. No doubt you'll want to create an announcement that reflects your personality.

Birth Announcement

Alexis and Chuck Dupree (especially Alexis) are pleased to announce the birth of Marie Curie Dupree, Alexis' right knee replacement.

"Thank God for Marie Curie!" Alexis said. "It's been a long metaphorical pregnancy to reach the point of birth. We are now settling down to the physical accommodation phase of knee infancy. There's no cooing, cuddling, or cute baby clothes, just physical therapy and lots of ice while we get used to each other."

The Goddess, Alexis' alter ego, will help Alexis during the first weeks or months of infancy. Chuck's mom, Marcelle Dupree, is also coming to assist. She is, after all, the proud grandmother of Marie Curie. No doubt her own relatively new knees will welcome Marie into the trending knee replacement community.

Born: June 10, 2014, around 9:30 a.m.
Where: Circa Hospital, Nearme, Mystate

Birth

Birth Announcement

Use this page to craft the birth announcement for your new knee:

_____

_____

_____

_____

_____

_____

_____

_____

_____

_____

_____

_____

_____

_____

_____

_____

_____

_____

_____

_____

_____

_____

_____

_____

_____

Birth

Birth Announcement

Use this page to craft the birth announcement for your new knee:

_____

_____

_____

_____

_____

_____

_____

_____

_____

_____

_____

_____

_____

_____

_____

_____

_____

_____

_____

_____

_____

_____

_____

_____

_____

_____

_____

_____

Birth

B

Recovery Journal

This appendix is divided into the following sections:

- "Appointments" on page 78—Keep a list of all of your medical and physical therapy appointsments in this section.

- "Medicines" on page 86—List all of your medicines and the frequency with which you need to take them in this section.

- "Medical Log" on page 88—Use this section each day to record the specific time you take medication.

Remember: Surgery can make you tired and forgetful. Pain does the same thing. A schedule of when you take the medicines, especially pain medicine, helps prevent problems.

- "Journal" on page 96—Keep a day-to-day journal of your recovery, notes to ask your surgeon or nursing staff or your physical therapist, and record your mood or pain level.

Appointments

Record any upcoming medical or physical therapy appointments
in this table.

Date	Time	Appointment

Appointments

Record any upcoming medical or physical therapy appointments in this table.

Date	Time	Appointment

Appointments

Record any upcoming medical or physical therapy appointments
in this table.

Appointments (side tab)

Date	Time	Appointment

Appointments

Record any upcoming medical or physical therapy appointments in this table.

Date	Time	Appointment

Appointments

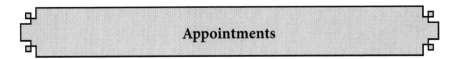

Appointments

Record any upcoming medical or physical therapy appointments in this table.

Date	Time	Appointment

Appointments

Appointments

Record any upcoming medical or physical therapy appointments in this table.

Date	Time	Appointment

Appointments

Appointments

Record any upcoming medical or physical therapy appointments in this table.

Date	Time	Appointment

Appointments

Record any upcoming medical or physical therapy appointments in this table.

Date	Time	Appointment

Appointments

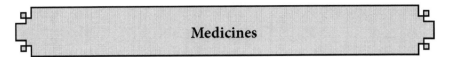

Medicines

Record all of your prescriptions, their dosage, and the frequency
with which you need to take them.

Prescription	Dosage	Frequency

Medicines

Medicines

Record all of your prescriptions, their dosage, and the frequency with which you need to take them.

Prescription	Dosage	Frequency
_____	_____	_____
_____	_____	_____
_____	_____	_____
_____	_____	_____
_____	_____	_____
_____	_____	_____
_____	_____	_____
_____	_____	_____
_____	_____	_____
_____	_____	_____
_____	_____	_____
_____	_____	_____
_____	_____	_____
_____	_____	_____
_____	_____	_____
_____	_____	_____
_____	_____	_____
_____	_____	_____
_____	_____	_____
_____	_____	_____

Medicines

Medical Log

Record the date and times you took each prescription in the following table.

Date	Time	Prescription

Medicine Log

Medical Log

Record the date and times you took each prescription in the following table.

Date	Time	Prescription

Medicine Log

Medical Log

Record the date and times you took each prescription in the
following table.

Date	Time	Prescription

Medicine Log

Medical Log

Record the date and times you took each prescription in the following table.

Date	Time	Prescription
_____	_____	_____
_____	_____	_____
_____	_____	_____
_____	_____	_____
_____	_____	_____
_____	_____	_____
_____	_____	_____
_____	_____	_____
_____	_____	_____
_____	_____	_____
_____	_____	_____
_____	_____	_____
_____	_____	_____
_____	_____	_____
_____	_____	_____
_____	_____	_____
_____	_____	_____
_____	_____	_____
_____	_____	_____
_____	_____	_____
_____	_____	_____

Medicine Log

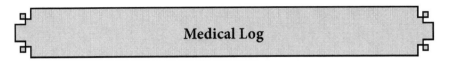

Medical Log

Record the date and times you took each prescription in the following table.

Date	Time	Prescription

Medicine Log

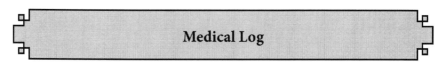

Medical Log

Record the date and times you took each prescription in the following table.

Date	Time	Prescription

Medicine Log

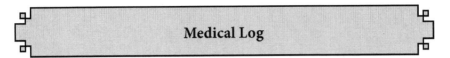

Medical Log

Record the date and times you took each prescription in the following table.

Date	Time	Prescription

Medicine Log

Medical Log

Record the date and times you took each prescription in the following table.

Date	Time	Prescription

Medicine Log

Date _____

Mood: _____ _____ Pain: 😞😐😊

_____
_____
_____
_____
_____
_____
_____
_____
_____
_____
_____
_____
_____
_____
_____
_____
_____
_____
_____
_____
_____
_____
_____
_____
_____
_____
_____

Journal

Date _____

Mood: _____ _____ Pain: ☹☺☺

_____
_____
_____
_____
_____
_____
_____
_____
_____
_____
_____
_____
_____
_____
_____
_____
_____
_____
_____
_____
_____
_____
_____
_____
_____

Journal

Date _____

Mood: _____ _____ Pain: ☹ 😐 ☺

_____
_____
_____
_____
_____
_____
_____
_____
_____
_____
_____
_____
_____
_____
_____
_____
_____
_____
_____
_____
_____
_____
_____
_____
_____
_____

Journal

Date _____

Mood: _____ Pain: ☹😐☺

_____
_____
_____
_____
_____
_____
_____
_____
_____
_____
_____
_____
_____
_____
_____
_____
_____
_____
_____
_____
_____
_____
_____
_____
_____
_____
_____
_____

Journal

Date _____

Mood: _____ _____ Pain: ☹😐☺

_____
_____
_____
_____
_____
_____
_____
_____
_____
_____
_____
_____
_____
_____
_____
_____
_____
_____
_____
_____
_____
_____
_____
_____

Journal

Date _____

Mood: _____ _____ Pain: ☹ 😐 ☺

_____

_____

_____

_____

_____

_____

_____

_____

_____

_____

_____

_____

_____

_____

_____

_____

_____

_____

Journal

_____

_____

_____

_____

_____

_____

_____

_____

Date _____

Mood: _____ _____ Pain: ☹☺☺

_____
_____
_____
_____
_____
_____
_____
_____
_____
_____
_____
_____
_____
_____
_____

Journal

_____
_____
_____
_____
_____
_____
_____
_____
_____

Date _____

Mood: _____ _____ Pain: ☹ 😐 ☺

_____
_____
_____
_____
_____
_____
_____
_____
_____
_____
_____
_____
_____
_____
_____
_____
_____
_____
_____
_____
_____
_____
_____
_____
_____
_____
_____
_____

Journal

Date _____

Mood: _____ _____ Pain: ☹ 😐 ☺

_____

_____

_____

_____

_____

_____

_____

_____

_____

_____

_____

_____

_____

_____

_____

Journal

_____

_____

_____

_____

_____

_____

_____

_____

_____

_____

_____

Date _____

Mood: _____ _____ Pain: ☹😐☺

_____
_____
_____
_____
_____
_____
_____
_____
_____
_____
_____
_____
_____
_____
_____
_____
_____
_____
_____
_____
_____
_____
_____
_____
_____
_____
_____
_____

Journal

Date _____

Mood: _____ _____ Pain: ☹ 😐 ☺

_____
_____
_____
_____
_____
_____
_____
_____
_____
_____
_____
_____
_____
_____
_____
_____
_____
_____

Journal

_____
_____
_____
_____
_____
_____
_____
_____
_____

Date _____

Mood: _____ _____ Pain: ☹ 😐 ☺

_____

_____

_____

_____

_____

_____

_____

_____

_____

_____

_____

_____

_____

_____

_____

_____

_____

Journal

_____

_____

_____

_____

_____

_____

_____

_____

Date _____

Mood: _____ _____ Pain: 😞😐😊

_____
_____
_____
_____
_____
_____
_____
_____
_____
_____
_____
_____
_____
_____
_____

Journal

_____
_____
_____
_____
_____
_____
_____
_____
_____

Date _____

Mood: _____ Pain: ☹☺☺

_____
_____
_____
_____
_____
_____
_____
_____
_____
_____
_____
_____
_____
_____
_____
_____
_____
_____
_____
_____
_____
_____
_____
_____
_____
_____
_____
_____

Journal

Date _____

Mood: _____ _____ Pain: ☹☺☺

_____
_____
_____
_____
_____
_____
_____
_____
_____
_____
_____
_____
_____
_____
_____
_____
_____
_____
_____
_____
_____
_____
_____
_____
_____
_____
_____
_____

Journal

Date _____

Mood: _____ _____ Pain: ☹😐☺

_____
_____
_____
_____
_____
_____
_____
_____
_____
_____
_____
_____
_____
_____
_____
_____
_____
_____
_____
_____
_____
_____
_____
_____
_____
_____
_____

Journal

Date _____

Mood: _____ _____ Pain: ☹😐☺

_____
_____
_____
_____
_____
_____
_____
_____
_____
_____
_____
_____
_____
_____
_____
_____
_____
_____

Journal

_____
_____
_____
_____
_____
_____
_____
_____
_____
_____

Date _____

Mood: _____ _____ Pain: ☹😐☺

_____
_____
_____
_____
_____
_____
_____
_____
_____
_____
_____
_____
_____
_____
_____
_____
_____
_____
_____
_____
_____
_____
_____
_____
_____
_____

Journal

Date _____

Mood: _____ _____ Pain: ☹ 😐 ☺

Date _____

Mood: _____ _____ Pain: ☹ 😐 ☺

_____
_____
_____
_____
_____
_____
_____
_____
_____
_____
_____
_____
_____
_____
_____
_____
_____
_____
_____
_____
_____
_____
_____
_____
_____
_____

Journal

Date _____

Mood: _____ _____ Pain: ☹ 😐 ☺

_____
_____
_____
_____
_____
_____
_____
_____
_____
_____
_____
_____
_____
_____
_____
_____
_____
_____
_____
_____
_____
_____
_____
_____
_____
_____
_____

Journal

Date _____

Mood: _____ _____ Pain: ☹😐☺

_____
_____
_____
_____
_____
_____
_____
_____
_____
_____
_____
_____
_____
_____
_____
_____
_____
_____
_____
_____
_____
_____
_____
_____
_____

Journal

Date _____

Mood: _____ _____ Pain: ☹😐☺

_____
_____
_____
_____
_____
_____
_____
_____
_____
_____
_____
_____
_____
_____
_____
_____
_____
_____
_____
_____
_____
_____
_____
_____
_____
_____

Journal

Date _____

Mood: _____ _____ Pain: ☹ 😐 ☺

_____
_____
_____
_____
_____
_____
_____
_____
_____
_____
_____
_____
_____
_____
_____
_____
_____
_____
_____
_____
_____
_____
_____
_____
_____
_____
_____

Journal

Date _____

Mood: _____ _____ Pain: ☹☺☺

_____
_____
_____
_____
_____
_____
_____
_____
_____
_____
_____
_____
_____
_____
_____

Journal

_____
_____
_____
_____
_____
_____
_____
_____
_____

Date _____

Mood: _____ _____ Pain: ☹😐☺

_____
_____
_____
_____
_____
_____
_____
_____
_____
_____
_____
_____
_____
_____
_____
_____
_____
_____
_____
_____
_____
_____
_____
_____
_____
_____

Journal

Date _____

Mood: _____ _____ Pain: ☹ 😐 ☺

_____
_____
_____
_____
_____
_____
_____
_____
_____
_____
_____
_____
_____
_____
_____
_____
_____
_____
_____
_____
_____
_____
_____
_____
_____
_____
_____
_____

Journal

Date _____

Mood: _____ _____ Pain: ☹😐☺

_____
_____
_____
_____
_____
_____
_____
_____
_____
_____
_____
_____
_____
_____
_____
_____
_____
_____
_____
_____
_____
_____
_____
_____
_____
_____
_____

Journal

Date _____

Mood: _____ _____ Pain: ☹ 😐 ☺

_____

_____

_____

_____

_____

_____

_____

_____

_____

_____

_____

_____

_____

_____

_____

Journal

_____

_____

_____

_____

_____

_____

_____

_____

_____

_____

Date _____

Mood: _____ _____ Pain: ☹😐☺

_____
_____
_____
_____
_____
_____
_____
_____
_____
_____
_____
_____
_____
_____
_____
_____
_____
_____
_____
_____
_____
_____
_____
_____
_____
_____
_____
_____
_____

Journal

Date _____

Mood: _____ _____ Pain: ☹😐☺

_____
_____
_____
_____
_____
_____
_____
_____
_____
_____
_____
_____
_____
_____

Journal

_____
_____
_____
_____
_____
_____
_____
_____
_____
_____
_____
_____

Date _____

Mood: _____ Pain: ☹ 😐 ☺

_____
_____
_____
_____
_____
_____
_____
_____
_____
_____
_____
_____
_____
_____
_____
_____
_____
_____
_____
_____
_____
_____
_____
_____
_____
_____
_____

Journal

Date _____

Mood: _____ _____ Pain: 😞😐☺

_____
_____
_____
_____
_____
_____
_____
_____
_____
_____
_____
_____
_____
_____
_____
_____
_____
_____
_____
_____
_____
_____
_____
_____
_____
_____

Journal

Date _____

Mood: _____ Pain: ☹☺☺

_____
_____
_____
_____
_____
_____
_____
_____
_____
_____
_____
_____
_____
_____
_____
_____
_____
_____
_____
_____
_____
_____
_____
_____
_____

Journal

Date _____

Mood: _____ _____ Pain: ☹️😐🙂

_____
_____
_____
_____
_____
_____
_____
_____
_____
_____
_____
_____
_____
_____
_____
_____

Journal

_____
_____
_____
_____
_____
_____
_____
_____
_____

Date _____

Mood: _____ Pain: ☹☺☺

_____

_____

_____

_____

_____

_____

_____

_____

_____

_____

_____

_____

_____

_____

_____

_____

_____

_____

Journal

_____

_____

_____

_____

_____

_____

_____

_____

Date _____

Mood: _____ _____ Pain: ☹😐☺

_____
_____
_____
_____
_____
_____
_____
_____
_____
_____
_____
_____
_____
_____
_____
_____
_____
_____
_____
_____
_____
_____
_____
_____
_____

Journal

Date _____

Mood: _____ _____ Pain: ☹😐☺

_____

_____

_____

_____

_____

_____

_____

_____

_____

_____

_____

_____

_____

_____

_____

_____

_____

_____

_____

_____

_____

_____

_____

_____

_____

Journal

Date _____

Mood: _____ Pain: 😞😐😊

_____
_____
_____
_____
_____
_____
_____
_____
_____
_____
_____
_____
_____
_____
_____

Journal

_____
_____
_____
_____
_____
_____
_____
_____
_____
_____
_____

Date _____

Mood: _____ _____ Pain: 😞😐😊

_____
_____
_____
_____
_____
_____
_____
_____
_____
_____
_____
_____
_____
_____
_____
_____
_____
_____
_____
_____
_____
_____
_____
_____
_____
_____
_____
_____

Journal

Date _____

Mood: _____ Pain: ☹ 😐 ☺

_____
_____
_____
_____
_____
_____
_____
_____
_____
_____
_____
_____
_____
_____
_____
_____
_____
_____
_____
_____
_____
_____
_____
_____
_____
_____

Journal

Date _____

Mood: _____ _____ Pain: ☹😐☺

_____
_____
_____
_____
_____
_____
_____
_____
_____
_____
_____
_____
_____
_____
_____
_____
_____
_____
_____
_____
_____
_____
_____
_____
_____
_____
_____
_____

Journal

Date _____

Mood: _____ Pain: ☹ 😐 ☺

_____
_____
_____
_____
_____
_____
_____
_____
_____
_____
_____
_____
_____
_____
_____
_____
_____
_____
_____
_____
_____
_____
_____
_____

Journal

Date _____

Mood: _____ _____ Pain: ☹ 😐 ☺

_____
_____
_____
_____
_____
_____
_____
_____
_____
_____
_____
_____
_____
_____
_____
_____
_____
_____
_____
_____
_____
_____
_____
_____
_____
_____
_____
_____

Journal

Date _____

Mood: _____ Pain: ☹️😐🙂

_____
_____
_____
_____
_____
_____
_____
_____
_____
_____
_____
_____
_____
_____
_____
_____
_____
_____
_____
_____
_____
_____
_____
_____
_____
_____
_____

Journal

Date _____

Mood: _____ Pain: 😟😐😊

_____
_____
_____
_____
_____
_____
_____
_____
_____
_____
_____
_____
_____
_____
_____
_____
_____
_____
_____

Journal

_____
_____
_____
_____
_____
_____
_____
_____

Date _____

Mood: _____ _____ Pain: ☹ 😐 ☺

_____
_____
_____
_____
_____
_____
_____
_____
_____
_____
_____
_____
_____
_____
_____
_____
_____
_____

Journal

_____
_____
_____
_____
_____
_____
_____
_____
_____

Date _____

Mood: _____ Pain: ☹ 😐 ☺

_____
_____
_____
_____
_____
_____
_____
_____
_____
_____
_____
_____
_____
_____
_____
_____
_____
_____
_____
_____
_____
_____
_____
_____
_____
_____
_____
_____

Journal

Date _____

Mood: _____ Pain: ☹😐☺

_____
_____
_____
_____
_____
_____
_____
_____
_____
_____
_____
_____
_____
_____
_____
_____
_____
_____
_____
_____
_____
_____
_____
_____

Journal

Date _____

Mood: _____ _____ Pain: ☹😐☺

_____

_____

_____

_____

_____

_____

_____

_____

_____

_____

_____

_____

_____

_____

_____

_____

_____

_____

_____

_____

_____

_____

_____

_____

_____

_____

_____

Journal

Date _____

Mood: _____ _____ Pain: ☹☺☺

_____
_____
_____
_____
_____
_____
_____
_____
_____
_____
_____
_____
_____
_____
_____
_____
_____
_____
_____
_____
_____
_____
_____
_____
_____
_____
_____

Journal

Date _____

Mood: _____ _____ Pain: ☹😐☺

_____

_____

_____

_____

_____

_____

_____

_____

_____

_____

_____

_____

_____

_____

_____

_____

_____

_____

_____

_____

_____

_____

_____

_____

_____

Journal

Date _____

Mood: _____ _____ Pain: ☹ 😐 ☺

_____
_____
_____
_____
_____
_____
_____
_____
_____
_____
_____
_____
_____
_____
_____
_____
_____
_____
_____
_____
_____
_____
_____
_____
_____

Journal

Date _____

Mood: _____ _____ Pain: ☹😐☺

_____
_____
_____
_____
_____
_____
_____
_____
_____
_____
_____
_____
_____
_____
_____
_____
_____
_____

Journal

_____
_____
_____
_____
_____
_____
_____
_____
_____

Date _____

Mood: _____ _____ Pain: ☹ 😐 ☺

_____
_____
_____
_____
_____
_____
_____
_____
_____
_____
_____
_____
_____
_____
_____
_____
_____
_____
_____
_____
_____
_____
_____
_____
_____
_____
_____

Journal

Date _____

Mood: _____ Pain: ☹️😐🙂

_____
_____
_____
_____
_____
_____
_____
_____
_____
_____
_____
_____
_____
_____
_____
_____
_____

Journal

_____
_____
_____
_____
_____
_____
_____
_____
_____

Date _____

Mood: _____ _____ Pain: ☹😐☺

_____
_____
_____
_____
_____
_____
_____
_____
_____
_____
_____
_____
_____
_____
_____
_____
_____
_____
_____
_____
_____
_____
_____
_____
_____
_____

Journal

Date _____

Mood: _____ Pain: ☹☺☺

_____
_____
_____
_____
_____
_____
_____
_____
_____
_____
_____
_____
_____
_____
_____
_____
_____
_____

Journal

_____
_____
_____
_____
_____
_____
_____
_____
_____

Date _____

Mood: _____ _____ Pain: ☹☺☺

_____
_____
_____
_____
_____
_____
_____
_____
_____
_____
_____
_____
_____
_____
_____
_____
_____

Journal

_____
_____
_____
_____
_____
_____
_____
_____
_____
_____
_____

Date _____

Mood: _____ _____ Pain: ☹☺☺

_____
_____
_____
_____
_____
_____
_____
_____
_____
_____
_____
_____
_____
_____
_____
_____
_____
_____
_____
_____
_____
_____
_____
_____
_____
_____

Journal

Date _____

Mood: _____ _____ Pain: ☹ 😐 ☺

_____
_____
_____
_____
_____
_____
_____
_____
_____
_____
_____
_____
_____
_____
_____
_____
_____
_____
_____
_____
_____
_____
_____
_____

Journal

Date _____

Mood: _____ Pain: ☹ 😐 ☺

_____
_____
_____
_____
_____
_____
_____
_____
_____
_____
_____
_____
_____
_____
_____
_____
_____
_____
_____
_____
_____
_____
_____
_____
_____
_____
_____

Journal

Date _____

Mood: _____ _____ Pain: ☹☺☺

_____

_____

_____

_____

_____

_____

_____

_____

_____

_____

_____

_____

_____

_____

_____

_____

_____

_____

_____

_____

_____

_____

Journal

_____

_____

_____

_____

_____

_____

_____

Date _____

Mood: _____ _____ Pain: ☹ 😐 ☺

_____
_____
_____
_____
_____
_____
_____
_____
_____
_____
_____
_____
_____
_____
_____
_____
_____
_____
_____
_____
_____
_____
_____
_____
_____
_____
_____
_____
_____

Journal

Date _____

Mood: _____ _____ Pain: ☹ 😐 ☺

_____
_____
_____
_____
_____
_____
_____
_____
_____
_____
_____
_____
_____
_____
_____

Journal

_____
_____
_____
_____
_____
_____
_____
_____
_____

Date _____

Mood: _____ Pain: ☹ 😐 ☺

_____
_____
_____
_____
_____
_____
_____
_____
_____
_____
_____
_____
_____
_____
_____
_____
_____
_____
_____
_____
_____
_____
_____
_____
_____
_____

Journal

Date _____

Mood: _____ Pain: ☹ 😐 ☺

_____
_____
_____
_____
_____
_____
_____
_____
_____
_____
_____
_____
_____
_____
_____
_____
_____
_____
_____
_____
_____
_____
_____
_____
_____

Journal

Date _____

Mood: _____ Pain: ☹😐☺

_____
_____
_____
_____
_____
_____
_____
_____
_____
_____
_____
_____
_____
_____
_____
_____
_____
_____
_____
_____
_____
_____
_____
_____
_____
_____

Journal

Date _____

Mood: _____ _____ Pain: ☹️😐🙂

_____
_____
_____
_____
_____
_____
_____
_____
_____
_____
_____
_____
_____
_____

Journal

_____
_____
_____
_____
_____
_____
_____
_____
_____

Date _____

Mood: _____ Pain: ☹ 😐 ☺

_____
_____
_____
_____
_____
_____
_____
_____
_____
_____
_____
_____
_____
_____
_____
_____
_____
_____
_____
_____
_____
_____
_____
_____
_____
_____
_____

Journal

Date _____

Mood: _____ Pain: ☹️😐🙂

_____
_____
_____
_____
_____
_____
_____
_____
_____
_____
_____
_____
_____
_____
_____
_____
_____
_____

Journal

_____
_____
_____
_____
_____
_____
_____
_____
_____

Date _____

Mood: _____ _____ Pain: ☹ 😐 ☺

_____
_____
_____
_____
_____
_____
_____
_____
_____
_____
_____
_____
_____
_____
_____
_____
_____
_____
_____
_____
_____
_____
_____
_____
_____
_____

Journal

Date _____

Mood: _____ _____ Pain: ☹ 😐 ☺

_____
_____
_____
_____
_____
_____
_____
_____
_____
_____
_____
_____
_____
_____
_____
_____
_____
_____
_____
_____
_____
_____
_____
_____
_____
_____
_____

Journal

Date _____

Mood: _____ _____ Pain: ☹😐☺

_____

_____

_____

_____

_____

_____

_____

_____

_____

_____

_____

_____

_____

_____

_____

_____

_____

_____

_____

_____

_____

_____

_____

_____

_____

_____

_____

Journal

Date _____

Mood: _____ Pain: ☹☺☺

_____
_____
_____
_____
_____
_____
_____
_____
_____
_____
_____
_____
_____
_____
_____
_____
_____

Journal

_____
_____
_____
_____
_____
_____
_____
_____
_____
_____
_____

Date _____

Mood: _____ _____ Pain: ☹😐☺

_____
_____
_____
_____
_____
_____
_____
_____
_____
_____
_____
_____
_____
_____
_____
_____
_____
_____
_____
_____
_____
_____
_____
_____
_____
_____
_____

Journal

Date _____

Mood: _____ _____ Pain: ☹ 😐 ☺

_____
_____
_____
_____
_____
_____
_____
_____
_____
_____
_____
_____
_____
_____
_____
_____
_____
_____
_____
_____
_____
_____
_____
_____
_____
_____

Journal

Date _____

Mood: _____ _____ Pain: ☹😐☺

_____
_____
_____
_____
_____
_____
_____
_____
_____
_____
_____
_____
_____
_____
_____
_____
_____
_____
_____
_____
_____
_____
_____
_____
_____
_____
_____

Journal

Date _____

Mood: _____ Pain: ☹😐☺

_____
_____
_____
_____
_____
_____
_____
_____
_____
_____
_____
_____
_____
_____
_____
_____
_____
_____
_____
_____
_____
_____
_____
_____

Journal

Date _____

Mood: _____ Pain: ☹ 😐 ☺

_____
_____
_____
_____
_____
_____
_____
_____
_____
_____
_____
_____
_____
_____
_____
_____
_____
_____
_____
_____
_____
_____
_____
_____
_____
_____
_____
_____
_____
_____
_____

Journal

Date _____

Mood: _____ _____ Pain: ☹☺☺

_____
_____
_____
_____
_____
_____
_____
_____
_____
_____
_____
_____
_____
_____
_____
_____

Journal

_____
_____
_____
_____
_____
_____
_____
_____
_____
_____
_____

Date _____

Mood: _____ _____ Pain: ☹️😐🙂

_____
_____
_____
_____
_____
_____
_____
_____
_____
_____
_____
_____
_____
_____
_____
_____
_____
_____
_____
_____
_____
_____
_____
_____
_____
_____
_____

Journal

Date _____

Mood: _____ _____ Pain: ☹ 😐 ☺

_____
_____
_____
_____
_____
_____
_____
_____
_____
_____
_____
_____
_____
_____
_____
_____
_____
_____

Journal

_____
_____
_____
_____
_____
_____
_____
_____

Date _____

Mood: _____ Pain: ☹ 😐 ☺

_____
_____
_____
_____
_____
_____
_____
_____
_____
_____
_____
_____
_____
_____
_____
_____
_____
_____
_____
_____
_____
_____
_____
_____
_____
_____
_____

Journal

Date _____

Mood: _____ _____ Pain: ☹ 😐 ☺

_____
_____
_____
_____
_____
_____
_____
_____
_____
_____
_____
_____
_____
_____
_____
_____
_____

Journal

_____
_____
_____
_____
_____
_____
_____
_____
_____
_____
_____

Date _____

Mood: _____ Pain: ☹😐☺

_____
_____
_____
_____
_____
_____
_____
_____
_____
_____
_____
_____
_____
_____
_____
_____
_____
_____
_____
_____
_____
_____
_____
_____
_____
_____
_____
_____
_____

Journal

Date _____

Mood: _____ Pain: ☹ 😐 ☺

_____
_____
_____
_____
_____
_____
_____
_____
_____
_____
_____
_____
_____
_____
_____
_____

Journal

_____
_____
_____
_____
_____
_____
_____
_____
_____

Date _____

Mood: _____ Pain: ☹ 😐 ☺

_____
_____
_____
_____
_____
_____
_____
_____
_____
_____
_____
_____
_____
_____
_____
_____
_____
_____
_____
_____
_____
_____
_____
_____
_____
_____
_____

Journal

Date _____

Mood: _____ _____ Pain: ☹️ 😐 🙂

_____
_____
_____
_____
_____
_____
_____
_____
_____
_____
_____
_____
_____
_____
_____
_____
_____
_____
_____
_____
_____
_____
_____
_____
_____
_____

Journal

Date _____

Mood: _____ Pain: ☹ 😐 ☺

_____
_____
_____
_____
_____
_____
_____
_____
_____
_____
_____
_____
_____
_____
_____
_____
_____
_____
_____
_____
_____
_____
_____
_____
_____
_____

Journal

Date _____

Mood: _____ _____ Pain: ☹☺☺

_____
_____
_____
_____
_____
_____
_____
_____
_____
_____
_____
_____
_____
_____
_____
_____
_____

Journal

_____
_____
_____
_____
_____
_____
_____
_____
_____
_____
_____

Date _____

Mood: _____ _____ Pain: 😞😐😊

_____
_____
_____
_____
_____
_____
_____
_____
_____
_____
_____
_____
_____
_____
_____
_____
_____
_____
_____
_____
_____
_____
_____
_____
_____
_____
_____
_____

Journal

Date _____

Mood: _____ _____ Pain: ☹😐☺

_____
_____
_____
_____
_____
_____
_____
_____
_____
_____
_____
_____
_____
_____
_____
_____
_____
_____
_____
_____
_____
_____
_____
_____
_____

Journal

Date _____

Mood: _____ Pain: ☹ 😐 ☺

_____
_____
_____
_____
_____
_____
_____
_____
_____
_____
_____
_____
_____
_____
_____
_____
_____
_____
_____
_____
_____
_____
_____
_____
_____
_____
_____

Journal

Date _____

Mood: _____ Pain: ☹😐☺

_____
_____
_____
_____
_____
_____
_____
_____
_____
_____
_____
_____
_____
_____

Journal

_____
_____
_____
_____
_____
_____
_____
_____
_____

Date _____

Mood: _____ _____ Pain: ☹ 😐 ☺

_____
_____
_____
_____
_____
_____
_____
_____
_____
_____
_____
_____
_____
_____
_____
_____
_____
_____
_____
_____
_____
_____
_____
_____
_____
_____

Journal

Date _____

Mood: _____ Pain: ☹ 😐 ☺

_____
_____
_____
_____
_____
_____
_____
_____
_____
_____
_____
_____
_____
_____
_____
_____
_____
_____
_____
_____
_____
_____
_____
_____
_____

Journal

Date _____

Mood: _____ _____ Pain: ☹ 😐 ☺

_____
_____
_____
_____
_____
_____
_____
_____
_____
_____
_____
_____
_____
_____
_____
_____
_____
_____
_____
_____
_____
_____
_____
_____
_____
_____

Journal

Date _____

Mood: _____ Pain: ☹ 😐 ☺

_____
_____
_____
_____
_____
_____
_____
_____
_____
_____
_____
_____
_____
_____
_____
_____

Journal

_____
_____
_____
_____
_____
_____
_____
_____
_____
_____
_____

Date _____

Mood: _____ Pain: ☹ 😐 ☺

_____
_____
_____
_____
_____
_____
_____
_____
_____
_____
_____
_____
_____
_____
_____
_____
_____
_____
_____

Journal

_____
_____
_____
_____
_____
_____
_____

Date _____

Mood: _____ _____ Pain: ☹ 😐 ☺

_____

_____

_____

_____

_____

_____

_____

_____

_____

_____

_____

_____

_____

_____

_____

Journal

_____

_____

_____

_____

_____

_____

_____

_____

_____

_____

Date _____

Mood: _____ _____ Pain: ☹ 😐 ☺

_____
_____
_____
_____
_____
_____
_____
_____
_____
_____
_____
_____
_____
_____
_____
_____
_____
_____
_____
_____
_____
_____
_____
_____
_____
_____
_____
_____

Journal

Date _____

Mood: _____ _____ Pain: ☹😐☺

_____
_____
_____
_____
_____
_____
_____
_____
_____
_____
_____
_____
_____
_____
_____

Journal

_____
_____
_____
_____
_____
_____
_____
_____
_____
_____
_____

Date _____

Mood: _____ Pain: ☹😐☺

_____
_____
_____
_____
_____
_____
_____
_____
_____
_____
_____
_____
_____
_____
_____
_____
_____
_____
_____
_____
_____
_____
_____
_____
_____
_____

Journal

Date _____

Mood: _____ Pain: ☹😐☺

_____

_____

_____

_____

_____

_____

_____

_____

_____

_____

_____

_____

_____

_____

_____

_____

_____

_____

_____

_____

_____

_____

_____

_____

_____

_____

Journal

Date _____

Mood: _____ Pain: ☹ 😐 ☺

_____
_____
_____
_____
_____
_____
_____
_____
_____
_____
_____
_____
_____
_____
_____
_____
_____
_____
_____
_____
_____
_____
_____
_____
_____
_____
_____
_____

Journal

Date _____

Mood: _____ _____ Pain: ☹ 😐 ☺

_____
_____
_____
_____
_____
_____
_____
_____
_____
_____
_____
_____
_____
_____
_____
_____
_____
_____
_____
_____
_____
_____
_____
_____
_____

Journal

Date _____

Mood: _____ _____ Pain: ☹ 😐 ☺

_____
_____
_____
_____
_____
_____
_____
_____
_____
_____
_____
_____
_____
_____
_____
_____
_____
_____
_____
_____
_____
_____
_____
_____
_____
_____

Journal

Date _____

Mood: _____ _____ Pain: ☹😐☺

_____
_____
_____
_____
_____
_____
_____
_____
_____
_____
_____
_____
_____
_____
_____
_____
_____
_____
_____
_____
_____
_____
_____
_____
_____

Journal

Date _____

Mood: _____ _____ Pain: ☹😐☺

_____
_____
_____
_____
_____
_____
_____
_____
_____
_____
_____
_____
_____
_____
_____
_____
_____
_____
_____
_____
_____
_____
_____
_____
_____
_____
_____
_____
_____
_____
_____
_____

Journal

Date _____

Mood: _____ _____ Pain: ☹😐☺

_____
_____
_____
_____
_____
_____
_____
_____
_____
_____
_____
_____
_____
_____
_____

Journal

_____
_____
_____
_____
_____
_____
_____
_____
_____

Date _____

Mood: _____ _____ Pain: ☹😐☺

_____
_____
_____
_____
_____
_____
_____
_____
_____
_____
_____
_____
_____
_____
_____
_____
_____
_____
_____
_____
_____
_____
_____
_____
_____
_____

Journal

Date _____

Mood: _____ _____ Pain: ☹😐☺

_____
_____
_____
_____
_____
_____
_____
_____
_____
_____
_____
_____
_____
_____
_____
_____

Journal

_____
_____
_____
_____
_____
_____
_____
_____
_____
_____

Date _____

Mood: _____ _____ Pain: ☹ 😐 ☺

_____

_____

_____

_____

_____

_____

_____

_____

_____

_____

_____

_____

_____

_____

_____

_____

_____

_____

_____

Journal

_____

_____

_____

_____

_____

_____

_____

_____

Date _____

Mood: _____ _____ Pain: ☹😐☺

_____
_____
_____
_____
_____
_____
_____
_____
_____
_____
_____
_____
_____
_____
_____
_____

Journal

_____
_____
_____
_____
_____
_____
_____
_____
_____

Date _____

Mood: _____ Pain: ☹ 😐 ☺

_____
_____
_____
_____
_____
_____
_____
_____
_____
_____
_____
_____
_____
_____
_____
_____
_____

Journal

_____
_____
_____
_____
_____
_____
_____

Date _____

Mood: _____ _____ Pain: ☹ 😐 ☺

_____
_____
_____
_____
_____
_____
_____
_____
_____
_____
_____
_____
_____
_____
_____
_____
_____
_____
_____
_____
_____
_____
_____
_____
_____
_____

Journal

Date _____

Mood: _____ Pain: ☹😐☺

_____
_____
_____
_____
_____
_____
_____
_____
_____
_____
_____
_____
_____
_____
_____
_____
_____
_____
_____
_____
_____
_____
_____
_____
_____
_____

Journal

Date _____

Mood: _____ _____ Pain: ☹😐☺

_____
_____
_____
_____
_____
_____
_____
_____
_____
_____
_____
_____
_____
_____
_____
_____
_____
_____
_____
_____
_____
_____
_____
_____
_____
_____

Journal

Date _____

Mood: _____ _____ Pain: ☹ 😐 ☺

_____
_____
_____
_____
_____
_____
_____
_____
_____
_____
_____
_____
_____
_____
_____
_____
_____
_____
_____
_____
_____
_____
_____
_____
_____
_____
_____
_____

Journal

Date _____

Mood: _____ _____ Pain: 😞😐😊

_____

_____

_____

_____

_____

_____

_____

_____

_____

_____

_____

_____

_____

_____

_____

_____

Journal

_____

_____

_____

_____

_____

_____

_____

_____

_____

Date _____

Mood: _____ _____ Pain: ☹ 😐 ☺

_____
_____
_____
_____
_____
_____
_____
_____
_____
_____
_____
_____
_____
_____
_____
_____
_____
_____
_____
_____
_____
_____
_____
_____
_____
_____

Journal

Date _____

Mood: _____ Pain: ☹ 😐 ☺

_____
_____
_____
_____
_____
_____
_____
_____
_____
_____
_____
_____
_____
_____
_____
_____
_____
_____
_____
_____
_____
_____
_____
_____
_____

Journal

Date _____

Mood: _____ _____ Pain: ☹😐☺

_____
_____
_____
_____
_____
_____
_____
_____
_____
_____
_____
_____
_____
_____
_____
_____
_____
_____
_____
_____
_____
_____
_____
_____
_____
_____
_____
_____
_____

Journal

Date _____

Mood: _____ _____ Pain: ☹ 😐 ☺

_____
_____
_____
_____
_____
_____
_____
_____
_____
_____
_____
_____
_____
_____
_____
_____
_____
_____
_____
_____
_____
_____
_____
_____
_____
_____
_____

Journal

Date _____

Mood: _____ _____ Pain: ☹😐☺

_____

_____

_____

_____

_____

_____

_____

_____

_____

_____

_____

_____

_____

_____

_____

_____

_____

_____

_____

Journal

_____

_____

_____

_____

_____

_____

_____

_____

Date _____

Mood: _____ Pain: ☹☺☺

_____
_____
_____
_____
_____
_____
_____
_____
_____
_____
_____
_____
_____
_____
_____
_____
_____
_____
_____
_____
_____
_____
_____
_____
_____

Journal

Date _____

Mood: _____ Pain: ☹ 😐 ☺

_____
_____
_____
_____
_____
_____
_____
_____
_____
_____
_____
_____
_____
_____
_____
_____
_____
_____
_____
_____
_____
_____
_____
_____
_____
_____

Journal

Date _____

Mood: _____ Pain: ☹ 😐 ☺

_____
_____
_____
_____
_____
_____
_____
_____
_____
_____
_____
_____
_____
_____
_____
_____
_____
_____
_____
_____
_____
_____
_____
_____
_____

Journal

Date _____

Mood: _____ _____ Pain: ☹ 😐 ☺

_____
_____
_____
_____
_____
_____
_____
_____
_____
_____
_____
_____
_____
_____
_____
_____
_____
_____
_____
_____
_____
_____
_____
_____
_____
_____
_____
_____

Journal

Date _____

Mood: _____ Pain: ☹😐☺

_____
_____
_____
_____
_____
_____
_____
_____
_____
_____
_____
_____
_____
_____
_____
_____
_____
_____
_____
_____
_____
_____
_____
_____
_____
_____

Journal

Date _____

Mood: _____ _____ Pain: ☹ 😐 ☺

_____
_____
_____
_____
_____
_____
_____
_____
_____
_____
_____
_____
_____
_____
_____
_____
_____
_____
_____
_____
_____
_____
_____
_____
_____
_____
_____

Journal

Date _____

Mood: _____ ____ Pain: ☹ 😐 ☺

_____
_____
_____
_____
_____
_____
_____
_____
_____
_____
_____
_____
_____
_____

Journal

_____
_____
_____
_____
_____
_____
_____
_____
_____
_____
_____

Date _____

Mood: _____ _____ Pain: ☹☺☺

_____
_____
_____
_____
_____
_____
_____
_____
_____
_____
_____
_____
_____
_____
_____
_____
_____
_____
_____
_____
_____
_____
_____
_____
_____
_____
_____

Journal

Date _____

Mood: _____ _____ Pain: ☹ 😐 ☺

_____
_____
_____
_____
_____
_____
_____
_____
_____
_____
_____
_____
_____
_____
_____
_____
_____
_____
_____
_____
_____
_____
_____
_____
_____

Journal

Date _____

Mood: _____ _____ Pain: ☹☺☺

_____
_____
_____
_____
_____
_____
_____
_____
_____
_____
_____
_____
_____
_____
_____
_____
_____
_____
_____

Journal

_____
_____
_____
_____
_____
_____
_____

Date _____

Mood: _____ _____ Pain: ☹ 😐 ☺

_____
_____
_____
_____
_____
_____
_____
_____
_____
_____
_____
_____
_____
_____
_____
_____
_____
_____
_____
_____
_____
_____
_____
_____
_____
_____
_____

Journal

Date _____

Mood: _____ Pain: 😟😐🙂

_____
_____
_____
_____
_____
_____
_____
_____
_____
_____
_____
_____
_____
_____
_____
_____
_____
_____
_____
_____
_____
_____
_____
_____
_____
_____
_____

Journal

Date _____

Mood: _____ _____ Pain: ☹😐☺

_____
_____
_____
_____
_____
_____
_____
_____
_____
_____
_____
_____
_____
_____
_____

Journal

_____
_____
_____
_____
_____
_____
_____
_____
_____

Date _____

Mood: _____ Pain: ☹ 😐 ☺

_____
_____
_____
_____
_____
_____
_____
_____
_____
_____
_____
_____
_____
_____
_____
_____
_____
_____
_____
_____
_____
_____
_____
_____
_____
_____
_____
_____

Journal

Date _____

Mood: _____ _____ Pain: ☹☺☺

_____
_____
_____
_____
_____
_____
_____
_____
_____
_____
_____
_____
_____
_____
_____
_____
_____
_____
_____
_____
_____
_____
_____
_____
_____
_____
_____

Journal

Date _____

Mood: _____ _____ Pain: ☹😐☺

_____
_____
_____
_____
_____
_____
_____
_____
_____
_____
_____
_____
_____
_____
_____
_____
_____
_____
_____
_____
_____
_____
_____
_____
_____
_____
_____

Journal

Date _____

Mood: _____ _____ Pain: ☹😐☺

_____
_____
_____
_____
_____
_____
_____
_____
_____
_____
_____
_____
_____
_____
_____
_____
_____

Journal

_____
_____
_____
_____
_____
_____
_____
_____
_____

Date _____

Mood: _____ Pain: 😦😐😊

_____

_____

_____

_____

_____

_____

_____

_____

_____

_____

_____

_____

_____

_____

_____

_____

_____

_____

_____

_____

_____

_____

_____

_____

Journal

Date _____

Mood: _____ _____ Pain: ☹ 😐 ☺

_____
_____
_____
_____
_____
_____
_____
_____
_____
_____
_____
_____
_____
_____
_____
_____
_____

Journal

_____
_____
_____
_____
_____
_____
_____
_____
_____

Date _____

Mood: _____ _____ Pain: ☹ 😐 ☺

_____
_____
_____
_____
_____
_____
_____
_____
_____
_____
_____
_____
_____
_____
_____
_____
_____
_____
_____
_____
_____
_____
_____
_____
_____
_____

Journal

Date _____

Mood: _____ _____ Pain: ☹️😐🙂

_____
_____
_____
_____
_____
_____
_____
_____
_____
_____
_____
_____
_____
_____
_____
_____
_____

Journal

_____
_____
_____
_____
_____
_____
_____
_____
_____

Date _____

Mood: _____ Pain: ☹ 😐 ☺

_____

_____

_____

_____

_____

_____

_____

_____

_____

_____

_____

_____

_____

_____

_____

_____

_____

_____

Journal

_____

_____

_____

_____

_____

_____

_____

_____

Date _____

Mood: _____ Pain: ☹😐☺

_____
_____
_____
_____
_____
_____
_____
_____
_____
_____
_____
_____
_____
_____
_____
_____

Journal

_____
_____
_____
_____
_____
_____
_____
_____
_____
_____

Date _____

Mood: _____ _____ Pain: ☹ 😐 ☺

_____
_____
_____
_____
_____
_____
_____
_____
_____
_____
_____
_____
_____
_____
_____
_____
_____
_____
_____
_____
_____
_____
_____
_____
_____

Journal

Date _____

Mood: _____ Pain: ☹ 😐 ☺

_____
_____
_____
_____
_____
_____
_____
_____
_____
_____
_____
_____
_____
_____
_____
_____

Journal

_____
_____
_____
_____
_____
_____
_____
_____
_____
_____

Date _____

Mood: _____ Pain: ☹ 😐 ☺

_____
_____
_____
_____
_____
_____
_____
_____
_____
_____
_____
_____
_____
_____
_____
_____
_____
_____
_____
_____
_____
_____
_____
_____
_____
_____
_____
_____

Journal

Date _____

Mood: _____ _____ Pain: ☹ 😐 ☺

_____
_____
_____
_____
_____
_____
_____
_____
_____
_____
_____
_____
_____
_____
_____
_____
_____
_____
_____
_____
_____
_____
_____
_____
_____
_____

Journal

Date _____

Mood: _____ _____ Pain: 😟😐😊

_____

_____

_____

_____

_____

_____

_____

_____

_____

_____

_____

_____

_____

_____

_____

_____

_____

_____

_____

_____

_____

_____

_____

_____

Journal

Date _____

Mood: _____ _____ Pain: ☹😐☺

_____

_____

_____

_____

_____

_____

_____

_____

_____

_____

_____

_____

_____

_____

Journal

_____

_____

_____

_____

_____

_____

_____

_____

_____

_____

Date _____

Mood: _____ _____ Pain: ☹☺☺

_____
_____
_____
_____
_____
_____
_____
_____
_____
_____
_____
_____
_____
_____
_____
_____
_____
_____
_____
_____
_____
_____
_____
_____
_____
_____
_____

Journal

Date _____

Mood: _____ _____ Pain: ☹ 😐 ☺

_____
_____
_____
_____
_____
_____
_____
_____
_____
_____
_____
_____
_____
_____
_____
_____
_____
_____
_____
_____
_____
_____
_____
_____

Journal

Date _____

Mood: _____ _____ Pain: ☹😐☺

_____
_____
_____
_____
_____
_____
_____
_____
_____
_____
_____
_____
_____
_____
_____
_____
_____
_____
_____
_____
_____
_____
_____
_____
_____
_____

Journal

Date _____

Mood: _____ _____ Pain: ☹ 😐 ☺

_____
_____
_____
_____
_____
_____
_____
_____
_____
_____
_____
_____
_____
_____
_____
_____
_____
_____
_____
_____
_____
_____
_____
_____

Journal

Date _____

Mood: _____ _____ Pain: 😞😐😊

_____
_____
_____
_____
_____
_____
_____
_____
_____
_____
_____
_____
_____
_____
_____
_____
_____
_____
_____
_____
_____
_____
_____
_____
_____
_____
_____
_____

Journal

Date _____

Mood: _____ _____ Pain: ☹😐☺

_____
_____
_____
_____
_____
_____
_____
_____
_____
_____
_____
_____
_____
_____
_____
_____
_____
_____
_____
_____
_____
_____
_____
_____
_____
_____

Journal

Date _____

Mood: _____ _____ Pain: ☹☺☺

_____
_____
_____
_____
_____
_____
_____
_____
_____
_____
_____
_____
_____
_____
_____
_____
_____
_____
_____
_____
_____
_____
_____
_____
_____
_____
_____
_____

Journal

Date _____

Mood: _____ _____ Pain: ☹☺☺

_____

_____

_____

_____

_____

_____

_____

_____

_____

_____

_____

_____

_____

_____

_____

_____

_____

_____

Journal

_____

_____

_____

_____

_____

_____

_____

_____

_____

Date _____

Mood: _____ _____ Pain: ☹😐☺

_____

_____

_____

_____

_____

_____

_____

_____

_____

_____

_____

_____

_____

_____

_____

_____

_____

_____

_____

_____

_____

_____

_____

_____

_____

_____

_____

Journal

Date _____

Mood: _____ _____ Pain: ☹😐☺

_____
_____
_____
_____
_____
_____
_____
_____
_____
_____
_____
_____
_____
_____
_____
_____
_____
_____
_____
_____
_____
_____
_____
_____
_____

Journal

Date _____

Mood: _____ _____ Pain: ☹ 😐 ☺

_____

_____

_____

_____

_____

_____

_____

_____

_____

_____

_____

_____

_____

_____

_____

_____

_____

_____

_____

_____

_____

_____

_____

_____

Journal

Date _____

Mood: _____ Pain: ☹😐☺

_____
_____
_____
_____
_____
_____
_____
_____
_____
_____
_____
_____
_____
_____
_____
_____
_____
_____
_____
_____
_____
_____
_____
_____
_____
_____
_____
_____

Journal

Date _____

Mood: _____ _____ Pain: ☹😐☺

_____
_____
_____
_____
_____
_____
_____
_____
_____
_____
_____
_____
_____
_____
_____
_____
_____
_____
_____
_____
_____
_____
_____
_____
_____
_____
_____
_____
_____

Journal

Date _____

Mood: _____ _____ Pain: ☹ 😐 ☺

_____
_____
_____
_____
_____
_____
_____
_____
_____
_____
_____
_____
_____
_____
_____
_____
_____
_____
_____
_____
_____
_____
_____
_____
_____
_____

Journal

Date _____

Mood: _____ _____ Pain: ☹😐☺

_____
_____
_____
_____
_____
_____
_____
_____
_____
_____
_____
_____
_____
_____
_____
_____
_____
_____
_____
_____
_____
_____
_____
_____
_____
_____
_____
_____
_____

Journal

Date _____

Mood: _____ _____ Pain: ☹ 😐 ☺

_____
_____
_____
_____
_____
_____
_____
_____
_____
_____
_____
_____
_____
_____
_____
_____

Journal

_____
_____
_____
_____
_____
_____
_____
_____
_____
_____
_____
_____

Date _____

Mood: _____ _____ Pain: ☹ 😐 ☺

_____
_____
_____
_____
_____
_____
_____
_____
_____
_____
_____
_____
_____
_____
_____
_____
_____
_____
_____
_____
_____
_____
_____
_____
_____
_____
_____
_____

Journal

Date _____

Mood: _____ _____ Pain: ☹ 😐 ☺

_____
_____
_____
_____
_____
_____
_____
_____
_____
_____
_____
_____
_____
_____
_____
_____
_____
_____
_____
_____
_____
_____
_____
_____
_____
_____

Journal

Date _____

Mood: _____ _____ Pain: ☹ 😐 ☺

_____
_____
_____
_____
_____
_____
_____
_____
_____
_____
_____
_____
_____
_____
_____
_____
_____
_____
_____
_____
_____
_____
_____
_____
_____

Journal

Date _____

Mood: _____ _____ Pain: ☹ 😐 ☺

_____
_____
_____
_____
_____
_____
_____
_____
_____
_____
_____
_____
_____
_____
_____
_____
_____
_____
_____
_____
_____
_____
_____
_____
_____
_____

Journal

Date _____

Mood: _____ _____ Pain: ☹ 😐 ☺

_____
_____
_____
_____
_____
_____
_____
_____
_____
_____
_____
_____
_____
_____
_____
_____
_____
_____
_____
_____
_____
_____
_____
_____
_____
_____
_____
_____

Journal

Date _____

Mood: _____ _____ Pain: ☹☺☺

_____
_____
_____
_____
_____
_____
_____
_____
_____
_____
_____
_____
_____
_____
_____
_____
_____
_____
_____
_____
_____
_____
_____
_____
_____
_____

Journal

Date _____

Mood: _____ _____ Pain: ☹😐☺

_____
_____
_____
_____
_____
_____
_____
_____
_____
_____
_____
_____
_____
_____
_____
_____
_____
_____
_____
_____
_____
_____
_____
_____
_____
_____
_____

Journal

Date _____

Mood: _____ _____ Pain: ☹😐☺

_____
_____
_____
_____
_____
_____
_____
_____
_____
_____
_____
_____
_____
_____
_____
_____
_____
_____
_____
_____
_____
_____
_____
_____

Journal

Date _____

Mood: _____ _____ Pain: ☹ 😐 ☺

_____
_____
_____
_____
_____
_____
_____
_____
_____
_____
_____
_____
_____
_____
_____
_____
_____
_____
_____
_____
_____
_____
_____
_____
_____
_____
_____
_____

Journal

Date _____

Mood: _____ _____ Pain: ☹ 😐 ☺

_____
_____
_____
_____
_____
_____
_____
_____
_____
_____
_____
_____
_____
_____
_____
_____
_____
_____
_____
_____
_____
_____
_____
_____
_____

Journal

Date _____

Mood: _____ _____ Pain: ☹️😐🙂

_____

_____

_____

_____

_____

_____

_____

_____

_____

_____

_____

_____

_____

_____

_____

_____

_____

_____

_____

_____

_____

_____

_____

_____

_____

_____

_____

Journal

Date _____

Mood: _____ Pain: ☹️😐😊

_____
_____
_____
_____
_____
_____
_____
_____
_____
_____
_____
_____
_____
_____
_____
_____

Journal

_____
_____
_____
_____
_____
_____
_____
_____
_____
_____
_____

About the Author

Journalist Alexis Dupree was 61 when she found herself joining the knee replacement community. She's now waiting for the cartilage in her left knee to give up the ghost so she can become a double member. In this book she shares what she learned to help you prepare for and recover successfully from knee replacement surgery.

Made in the USA
Lexington, KY
27 April 2018